#74984-1/2

DREAMS AND DUE DILIGENCE

Till and McCulloch's Stem Cell Discovery and Legacy

JOE SORNBERGER

Dreams and Due Diligence

Till and McCulloch's Stem Cell Discovery and Legacy

UNIVERSITY OF TORONTO PRESS
Toronto Buffalo London

Toronto Buffalo London
www.utppublishing.com
Printed in Canada

ISBN 978-1-4426-4485-4

Printed on acid-free, 100% post-consumer recycled paper with vegetable-based inks.

Library and Archives Canada Cataloguing in Publication

Sornberger, Joe, 1952–
Dreams and due diligence : Till and McCulloch's stem cell discovery and legacy / Joe Sornberger.

Includes bibliographical references and index.
ISBN 978-1-4426-4485-4

1. McCulloch, Ernest A. (Ernest Armstrong). 2. Till, James E. (James Edgar). 3. Stem cells – Research – Canada. 4. Medical research personnel – Canada – Biographies. I. Title

QH588.S83S67 2011 616'.02774092271 C2011-904824-8

University of Toronto Press acknowledges the financial assistance to its publishing program of the Canada Council for the Arts and the Ontario Arts Council.

Canada Council for the Arts Conseil des Arts du Canada
ONTARIO ARTS COUNCIL
CONSEIL DES ARTS DE L'ONTARIO

University of Toronto Press acknowledges the financial support of the Government of Canada through the Canada Book Fund for its publishing activities.

Dedicated to the memory
of Ernest Armstrong 'Bun' McCulloch
(1926–2011)

Contents

THE CANADIAN STEM CELL FOUNDATION ix
FOREWORD xi
ACKNOWLEDGMENTS xvii

Introduction 3

Part One: Discovery

1 On a Sunday in 1960 9

2 After the A-Bomb, before the Beatles 12

3 The Impossible Partnership 19

Part Two: Development

4 A Bunch of Kids Having a Good Time 49

5 The Progeny 66

Part Three: Today and Tomorrow

6 Ethics, Hope, and Hype 85

7 The Evil Twin: The Cancer Stem Cell 99

8 The Beneficiary 105

9 The Future 115

10 Little Fame, No Nobel 126

Conclusion 133

NOTES 139
INDEX 145

Photos follow page 78

The Canadian Stem Cell Foundation

This book was made possible through the leadership and financial support of the Canadian Stem Cell Foundation. The Foundation would like to thank the Stem Cell Network for their generous support.

The Canadian Stem Cell Foundation champions the importance of stem cell science for the health of humanity. It unifies scientists, business and community leaders, and the public. It also provides education and builds the partnerships necessary to accelerate the speed at which research is translated into clinical applications and therapies for people everywhere.

The Foundation is intent on building Canada's role as a stem cell leader and innovator. Stem cells were first discovered in Canada, and dozens of the field's brightest minds have made ground-breaking contributions here. The world is now closer to treatments and cures never before imagined because of them.

By continuing to support their important work and training the next generation of scientists, we can move even closer, and build an entirely new industry, with a global scope, to serve all humanity.

The Canadian Stem Cell Foundation is an independent, registered charitable organization.

Charitable Registration Number: 82816 9128 RR0001
www.stemcellfoundation.ca

Foreword

There have been two great revolutions in science over the past 100 years – first physics and now biology. This book tells the story of a key part of the revolution in the biological sciences. Since the Second World War, no area of science has made such extraordinary progress and achieved so many landmark advances as rapidly as biomedical research. These advances have profoundly changed how we view life on this planet, our bodies, human health, and disease.

The revolution in the biological sciences has many signposts, but two are fundamental: first, the discovery in the 1940s and early 1950s that our genetic information is embodied in DNA and, furthermore, as shown by Watson and Crick, that DNA has a double-helical structure. The second fundamental advance was the discovery in the 1960s by Till and McCulloch of stem cells, the cells in our body that have the unique capacity of being able to replace throughout our lifetimes the diverse cell types whose lifespan is much shorter than our own lives. These two advances – the first in DNA science and genetic engineering and the second in stem cell biology – have opened the door to a new era in biology and medicine. And they have brought within our grasp the realistic goal that we will soon understand the intricate workings of the human body at both the genetic and cellular levels and that this understanding will lead to entirely new approaches to the treatment of diseases and conditions as different as cancer and spinal cord injury.

Unlike the DNA story, which has entered the common lexicon, stem cells have only recently received public attention with the controversy surrounding the use of human embryos to generate embryonic stem cells. What are stem cells and why do they matter? First, a little biology: while DNA is the blueprint that makes us who we are, it is just that – a blueprint. Like a blueprint for a building, our DNA is not the building itself. Buildings are made up of specialized architectural components – bricks, windows, etc. Similarly, our body is made up of billions of cells with distinct functions and properties. For example, the neurons in our brain are responsible for transmitting and receiving tiny electrical messages that enable us to think, remember, speak, and so on. And the cells in our blood are made up of many distinct cell types – red blood cells transport oxygen to our tissues, platelets are central to forming blood clots when we bleed, and lymphocytes (which themselves are made up of several distinct types) fight off infection by viruses, bacteria, and parasites.

Most of these specialized cells live only for a short period of time. Our red cells, for example, live for about 120 days or four months. Hence, they have to be continuously replaced for the eighty or so years that most of us now live. It's as if bricks were continuously falling off a building and magically being replaced by new bricks every four months. And we are not talking about one or two bricks a year: our body has to be able to make millions of new red blood cells every minute of every day throughout our lives!

How does this daily miracle happen? And how were the secrets of stem cells first discovered? That is the story of Jim Till and Ernest (Bun) McCulloch, told so well by Joe Sornberger in the following pages.

One of the good fortunes that I have had throughout my scientific career is a front-row seat to the stem cell story, first as a graduate student in Jim Till's lab in the 1960s and early 1970s, then as an independent scientist who contributed to advances in stem cell science in various ways, and then as a scientific leader in my role as President of Canada's federal funding agency for health research, the Canadian Institutes of Health Research (CIHR).

Like many undergraduates in mathematics, physics, and chemistry in the 1960s, I was aware that there were exciting things happening in biomedical research, although I wasn't sure what they were or how to learn about them. Through a bit of luck, I ended up in Jim Till's lab in 1968 (at Jim's insistence, I never called him Dr Till but Jim and hence will do so here). Including the other students and technicians in Jim's lab at the time as well as a similar sized group in Dr McCulloch's lab (again, we referred to Dr McCulloch as either Dr McCulloch or, if we had the courage, to his boyhood nickname, Bun), we constituted the 'spleen team.'

As Joe Sornberger explains, the spleen team got its name from the properties of stem cells in mouse bone marrow; they could form colonies of millions of cells within seven to ten days – and, as Alan Wu and Andy Becker, graduate students in the spleen team showed, all descended from a single cell (the stem cell), on the spleens of mice that had been irradiated and then rescued with bone marrow cells from another mouse.

At Jim's insistence, the cells that gave rise to these colonies were not called stem cells but rather colony-forming units in the spleen (or CFU-S). This operational definition reflected Jim's approach to science – he insisted on an operational rather than a wishful but possibly incorrect definition. That rigour characterized all of the work of the spleen team: the operational definition of the stem cell, the elegant use of mouse genetics to show that the CFU-S was essential to blood cell production, and the chromosomal marker work has, to this day, been the gold standard for the stem cell research that has followed.

There were many lessons for the students who trained with Jim and Bun in those exciting days. First, Jim and Bun's success was based on collaboration between two individuals who couldn't have been more dissimilar. Their backgrounds, personality, training, and approach to science were as different as night and day: Jim was a product of the Canadian Prairies while Bun was the product of a solid Toronto private school upbringing. Jim received his PhD in biophysics from Yale, specializing in radiation biology, while Bun was a medical doctor specializing in hematology (blood cells) and leukemia. Where Jim is by nature conservative in his interpretation of data, Bun loved to speculate. And on a personal level, Jim was tall and athletic while Bun was short, balding, and more interested in books than the sport that Jim and most of the other scientific staff at the Ontario Cancer Institute loved – curling.

As students, we quickly appreciated that those differences were strengths and, coupled with complete trust and affection between the two men, were an unbeatable combination. Later, as president of CIHR, I thought often about Jim and Bun and the synergy that comes from collaboration.

Another lesson from the Toronto stem cell story is the unpredictability of science. Bun and Jim did not set out to find stem cells; indeed, I doubt whether Jim had even heard that term before! Rather, their task, urged on by Harold Johns – the father of medical biophysics at the OCI – was to answer a pressing problem in radiation treatment for cancer: determine a safe dose of radiation that could be delivered to a cancer patient, given the radiation sensitivity of normal cells, especially cells in the bone marrow. And so they set out to determine a way of measuring quantitatively the radiation sensitivity of bone marrow cells. In the course of doing that, they stumbled on the spleen colony-forming assay and stem cells. Their first paper was published in *Radiation Research*, a specialized journal that almost certainly no one interested in stem cells would ever read. And the title of that first paper, 'A Direct Measurement of the Radiation Sensitivity of Normal Mouse Bone Marrow Cells,' guaranteed that it would only be read by a very specialized, small audience. This story has stayed with me throughout my career: the directions and ultimate impact of science are unpredictable and therefore the best way to ensure relevance and impact is to focus on excellence.

Perhaps the most important lesson that I learned as Jim's student was his style of mentoring. When I joined the lab, there were already three other graduate students. Jim treated each of us differently, and as individuals. After a few months of working on blood stem cells, I decided that genetics was the key to biology. This conclusion was based on the beautiful experiments that Bun and Jim had done with Louis Siminovitch, then head of the Biology Division at the OCI and one of Canada's pre-eminent geneticists, and the group at the Bar Harbor Laboratory in Maine. By making use of naturally existing mouse mutants (*W* and *Steel*) that had defects in blood cell production, they showed that the *W* defect affected CFU-S directly and that *Steel* affected the cellular environment in which these cells live. When I read those papers in 1968, I was determined to understand the nature of the defects in these mutant mice. But that would require isolating the genes that encoded *W* and *Steel*, something that would only become possible years later with the advent of recombinant DNA technology. One of my greatest satisfactions as a scientist was when, twenty years later, Benoit Chabot, a postdoctoral fellow in my lab, and I isolated the *W* gene.

Jim let me pursue my own interests as a graduate student, and I switched projects from mouse stem cells to microbial genetics. When we would meet as student and mentor, we rarely discussed my science; rather, our discussions ranged from philosophy to the challenges Jim was having with some of the scientific staff in the Biology Division (by that time, Jim had succeeded Siminovitch as head).

Although I was not conscious of this at the time, I appreciated afterwards how Jim and Bun treated each student as their equal, expecting as much from us as they did from themselves. The discovery of stem cells is unquestionably an enormous legacy, but arguably an equally important legacy were the students who have gone on to make their own contributions to stem cell science and other areas of biomedical research. And, of course, over the past fifty years, that generation has now trained yet another generation of students. Many people today have written about the very real challenges facing young people in science. Jim and Bun understood fifty years ago the central importance of young people to biomedical research and the great contributions young people make to science.

The discovery of the hematopoietic (blood-forming) stem cell gradually began to receive wide attention over the next twenty years. That attention was greatly accelerated when human embryonic stem cells were isolated in the 1990s. These cells, unlike adult bone marrow cells, derive from early human embryos, raising simultaneously great hope that they have retained the capacity to give rise to *all* the cells in the human body and the ethical concern that such science will encourage the destruction of human embryos. When I became president of CIHR, one of the first things we did, therefore, was to put together a committee of scientists, ethicists, and lay people, chaired by Janet Rossant, a world-renowned developmental biologist and at the time my colleague at the Lunenfeld in Toronto, to advise CIHR's Governing Council on the policies that should oversee human embryonic stem cell research. Some members of Canada's Parliament objected strongly that CIHR was usurping Parliament's prerogative to set policy and legislation. However, CIHR's Governing Council wisely decided that, until such time as legislation was passed, CIHR had an obligation to develop and enforce guidelines to ensure that all research involving human embryos, and funded in whole or in part by CIHR, adhered to a set of guidelines that had been developed by reasonable and knowledgeable people. Now, almost a decade later, those guidelines have stood the test of time and served as a model for other countries, including the United States.

I tell this story to highlight another feature of the Till and McCulloch story – because of their contributions and their legacy of two generations of stem cell scientists, Canada has exceptional strength in stem cell science. If hockey is Canada's game, stem cell research is Canada's science. The discovery of neural stem cells, mesenchymal stem cells, and cancer stem cells, as well as important advances in human embryonic stem cell research, are all Canadian discoveries, as are important insights into the cellular and molecular aspects of human leukemia and other cancers. These scientific strengths extend into the ethical and policy areas around stem cells – Canadian scholars are recognized worldwide for their important contributions to these critical areas.

Let me conclude with a story: sometime in the early 1980s, Lloyd Old, then the distinguished president of the Ludwig Institute for Cancer Research based in New York, came to the OCI, then located on Sherbourne Street in Toronto, to look into establishing a branch of the Ludwig (which he did, led by Dr W.R. Bruce). At that time, the OCI occupied two floors of the Princess Margaret Hospital. After meeting with me in my office, Dr Old walked in front of me down the narrow, dingy hallway (narrow because of the centrifuges and ice machines that crammed the hallway) as I took him to his next appointment. Suddenly, he stopped, and, as I crashed into him, he looked around and said: 'What hallowed halls are these. To think that the stem cell was discovered here.' As I looked around, those old dingy hallways acquired a new significance: they were indeed hallowed hallways; the stem cell was indeed discovered there.

I hope that when you read this book you get the same sense of wonder and excitement that I still get when I think about the stem cell story – it is a Canadian story, a story of scientific discovery and of a new era in biomedical research, a story of two very different men who chose to work together, and in the end a story that has given more than hope for patients with cancer and other diseases.

A brief epilogue: the Nobel Committee has yet to recognize the pioneering work of Till and McCulloch, even though they are among the very few scientists who have received both Gairdner and Lasker awards, but not the Nobel. This oversight is unfortunate, especially as, sadly, Bun passed away during the fiftieth anniversary year of the discovery of the stem cell. Nevertheless, it is worth remembering that the discovery of insulin in Toronto in the 1920s (which was recognized with the Nobel Prize) and its use in the treatment of diabetes, followed by the discovery of stem cells in Toronto in the 1960s and the application of that discovery in the treatment of certain forms of cancer and anemias, stand today as landmarks in the use of a human protein and human cells, respectively, to treat disease.

Alan Bernstein, OC, PhD, FRSC, FCAHS

Acknowledgments

This book would not have been possible without the kind cooperation of James Edgar Till and Ernest Armstrong 'Bun' McCulloch.

Dr Till gave willingly of his time, sitting through interviews in which he patiently answered a layman's often-repeated, sometimes inane questions about the perplexing science he had helped found. He further contributed by reviewing the trickier science-based portions of the book to keep me from putting my foot too deeply in my mouth. He also helped in searching through old files, generously provided by the University of Toronto Archives, in the hope of finding elusive evidence of the partners' earliest experiments with their 'colony-forming units.'

Dr McCulloch, who was in failing health and nearing the end of his life while this book was being researched and written, also kindly agreed to be interviewed by telephone and in person, and his always sharp insights were invaluable. He died on 20 January 2011, when the last chapters of this book were still being written. Beyond the interview material he provided, his book, *The Ontario Cancer Institute – Successes and Reverses at Sherbourne Street* (McGill-Queen's University Press, 2003), proved to be a valuable resource and is referred to frequently in the pages that follow.

Many of the original Ontario Cancer Institute researchers also took the time to share their memories. Special thanks must go to Dr Lou Siminovitch, who worked closely with Drs Till and McCulloch, partnering with them on some of their most important papers. His self-published book, *Reflections on a Life in Science* (2003), was also a great help. As well, more than fifty leading scientists scattered across Canada, the United States, the United Kingdom, Europe, and Australia gave of their time to express their thoughts about Drs Till and McCulloch and the impact they had on their lives. These are people whose life's work is finding cures for cancer, spinal cord injury, and a host of degenerative diseases. Their time is exceedingly precious; I am grateful they were able to share some of it with me.

James Price of the Stem Cell Foundation deserves significant credit for suggesting that the Till and McCulloch story should be told in book form and for his expertly timed encouragement over several pad thai lunches. Thanks also to Eileen Emmonds at the foundation for her good-natured and tireless administrative help.

This book likely would not have been possible without Len Husband of the University of Toronto Press, who saw something worthwhile in the original all-over-the-place manuscript, helped restructure and refine it, and provided wise counsel during the revising process. Editor Matthew Kudelka greatly enhanced things with his elegant touch and keen eye, and Wayne Herrington deftly shepherded the pages through to publication. Jane Finlayson, at the University Health Network, also came through in a big way, especially in rounding up the archival photographs.

Closer to home, I want to thank my Bridgehead buddies Steve Judges, Don Gibbons, Jim Cocks, and Charles Hodgson for their constant support and unflagging friendship. And very special thanks go to my wife, Sue Michalicka, a much more gifted writer, whose encouragement and chocolate chip cookies make all things possible.

Finally, huge credit for what follows must go to my son, Michael Sornberger, who used breaks in his PhD studies at McGill University to do research, proof chapters, organize references, and offer insightful suggestions. I am a very fortunate father.

Joe Sornberger, Ottawa, June 2011

DREAMS AND DUE DILIGENCE

Till and McCulloch's Stem Cell Discovery and Legacy

Introduction

On the cover of a 2004 magazine produced by the Stem Cell Network, Ernest Armstrong McCulloch and James Edgar Till are pictured outside their offices at a railing overlooking the atrium at the Princess Margaret Hospital in Toronto. Till, with a full head of silver hair, smiles widely. McCulloch, bald, does not. They appear to be comparable in height, but this has been achieved by digitally lifting the image of the much smaller, stouter McCulloch to fit the frame better.

Tall and lean, short and stout. If physically they resembled Bert and Ernie come to life – or to go back further, Mutt and Jeff – they were just as dissimilar in personality. They had so little in common.

McCulloch was from Old Money Toronto and grew up in affluence with a private school education and a family place in the country. Belying his taciturn appearance, he had a million ideas running through his quick mind and would share them with anyone with a curious nature and the ability to keep up. He thought tangentially, constantly playing a game of connect the dots across many fields of interest. He could be funny and charming or witheringly caustic. He possessed a knowledge of literature not typically found in someone so passionate about science. 'He had a photographic memory as far as I could tell,' says a former close colleague. 'He seemed to remember everything he ever read. He could spout long, long pieces of poetry that he remembered from someplace.'

Till is no less quick of mind but far less likely to spout Shakespeare or trot out Trollope. He is more passionate about the physics of curling than the stories of Chekhov. A farmboy from Alberta, he collected enough academic prizes and scholarships in his youth to make it all the way to a Yale PhD and an offer of a position there, which he turned down for the chance to come back to Canada. Fittingly for a man with a facility for physics, mathematics, and statistics, he is known for presenting his ideas in a much more measured manner than his more unpredictable partner. He is often described as a straight arrow.

Together, they formed the most important partnership in Canadian medical research since Frederick Banting and Charles Best pooled their talents in the early 1920s and discovered insulin. Significantly, the discoveries that Till and McCulloch made may someday soon lead to daily insulin injections for diabetes becoming a thing of the past.

Unlike Banting and Best, however, Till and McCulloch remain largely unknown outside their field. While they have received almost every award available in medical research except for the Nobel, the general public has not heard about them. When McCulloch died in January 2011 at the age of eighty-four, Peter Mansbridge introduced the CBC News report by first explaining who the great man was. Had he been a hockey player or an actor in second-rate films, no such explanation would have been necessary. Such is the lot of a giant of medical research.

Till and McCulloch represent a great untold story. Their discovery of hematopoietic (blood-forming) stem cells stands as one of the most remarkable medical research achievements of the twentieth century. It came, as one distinguished leader in the field has said, 'like a bolt of lightning.' It opened up a whole new field of investigation: stem cell science.

They weren't alone, but part of a crew that helped set the course for cancer research in Canada and caused major reverberations around the world. At a time when Canada and Canadians tended to stand in the shadow of the United States, the United Kingdom, and Europe in terms of medical research, Till and McCulloch and their colleagues at the brand new Ontario Cancer Institute on Sherbourne Street in Toronto made many of the world's top researchers stop and change course.

Their legacy, however, is more than a collection of elegant papers that sparkle with genius. Till and McCulloch trained and influenced and inspired successive generations of medical researchers who have gone on to do great things. Some of the leading researchers in Canada and the world – people such as Tak Wah Mak and John Dick, Connie Eaves and Hans Messner – owe their success in large part to what they learned from or what was passed down from Till and McCulloch.

In terms of human health, thousands of people who would have died from leukemia and immunological diseases have gone on to live full and happy lives thanks to therapies developed from discoveries that

Till and McCulloch championed or because of advances made by subsequent generations of researchers. Their accomplishments were anything but arcane, and their impact has been very real and meaningful to many people.

So this is not a tale of two men tucked away in a lab, far removed from real life. This is the story of a discovery that spawned history-making changes in medicine and medical practice. This is the story of two men, as different as chalk and cheese, who shared a passion for scientific research and a dogged desire to succeed. They just happened to have exactly the right complementary talents to accomplish great things together. The whole truly was more than the sum of the parts.

It's a great story that, until now, has remained untold.

PART ONE

Discovery

1

On a Sunday in 1960

It must have been a cold day, because he would remember that the fireplace was crackling when he left the family home to head to the lab. He would recall the day 'vividly,' though he could no longer remember the date, except that it was a Sunday, or the season, though he thought it was autumn. But then, it would have been hard for anyone, let alone a man in his mid-eighties nearing the end of his life after several years of serious health problems, to retrieve a date from fifty years ago that wasn't a family birth, a wedding, or a death.

So let's agree that it was just an ordinary Sunday afternoon in 1960.

Ernest McCulloch went to work that day not to get away from his family – he had always adored his wife Ona, with whom he raised five children – and not because he was a workaholic, a term that would not be coined for several years. He was pulling a regular shift for any biology researcher: checking the specimens. It was the designated day to study the mice that he and research partner Jim Till had first exposed to full-body radiation, then injected with either irradiated or normal bone marrow cells. The idea was to assess radiation sensitivity, to see if injecting the already nuked mice with the nuked cells translated into changes in the kinds of cells found in the spleen – a prime location, along with bone marrow, for blood cell formation.

McCulloch's lab at the Ontario Cancer Institute (OCI) on Sherbourne Street was a five-minute drive from his home in the wealthy Toronto neighbourhood of Rosedale. The OCI has always been better known as the Princess Margaret Hospital, so named ostensibly to honour Queen Elizabeth's sister, who officially opened the building in 1958 – but more accurately to spare already ill patients the additional anxiety of entering a building with the word 'cancer' over its doors. The seven-storey building's top two floors were dedicated to research, with McCulloch's lab on the sixth floor and the mice in their cages on the floor above. That Sunday, he checked the mice's spleens, made some notes, and went back down to his office to try to make sense of it all.

Medical research experiments never really fail. The objective is to test a hypothesis. If the hypothesis proves true, with solid evidence to back it up, the experiment is a success. The new information gets published in a peer-reviewed journal and integrated into the circuitry of scientific knowledge. Maybe it helps to treat or even cure a disease. If the hypothesis proves false, the scientist at least has the satisfaction of ruling something out, crossing something off the list. It is still a success, but only sort of.

McCulloch's original plan was to test a hypothesis about possible differences in growth patterns between normal and irradiated blood-forming cells. On that Sunday, he was doing the work that needed to be done to test the hypothesis. And it was proving to be a sort-of success. As he would write in his book about the OCI, 'the experiment was successful in that the hypothesis on which it was based was disproved. No morphological difference was observed between intact and irradiated marrow; differentiation was not highly radiation-sensitive.'[1]

A lesser scientist might have called it a day and gone home to watch *The Ed Sullivan Show*. But something caught McCulloch's attention. The spleens of the mice that received the bone marrow injections had round, flesh-like bumps or nodules on them. He decided to count them and plot them on a graph. To his surprise, and considerable excitement, the number of the nodules, each of which it turned out was populated with proliferating blood cells, seemed to line up directly with the number of bone marrow cells the mouse had received. Suddenly, whether the original hypothesis was correct became far less interesting.

In the science of biology it had long been theorized that there was a single, original source that could replicate itself and transform into the cellular building material required to create, sustain, and repair the blood and bones, tissues and organs that make up a living body. But nobody had ever proved it.

Serendipity and scientific discovery often go hand-in-hand. In the 1840s, Charles Goodyear discovered how to vulcanize rubber when he dropped a piece of it on a stove. Alexander Fleming fluked his discovery of penicillin by leaving a dish of staphylococcus bacteria uncovered for a few days. But luck isn't enough in science. As Louis Pasteur maintained, 'In the fields of observation chance favors only the prepared mind.'[2]

On an ordinary Sunday in 1960, McCulloch sensed he had found the source.

The next day, McCulloch took the results to Till, who remembers him waving the paper excitedly. Even the normally unflappable Till got worked up. 'We knew it was something, yeah – something novel,' he would say fifty years later.

Within a year, in February 1961, Till and McCulloch published their findings in an innocuously titled paper – 'A Direct Measurement of the Radiation Sensitivity of Normal Mouse Bone Marrow Cells' – in a niche academic journal called *Radiation Research*.

It would change everything.

2

After the A-Bomb, before the Beatles

Toronto was a different place when James Till and Ernest McCulloch were setting to work on the paper that would change the way people thought about biology. While it had blossomed considerably from what McCulloch described as the 'miserable little town' he grew up in, it was a long way from the cosmopolitan centre it would become. There was no CN Tower or Rogers Centre. No Henry Moore sculpture on Nathan Phillips Square. The Toronto of 1960 was the kind of place where bars and movie theatres stayed shut on Sundays. If nothing short of world-class will do for Toronto today, fifty years ago it had a bad case of Buffalo envy.

Canada was also a very different country than it is today. While Americans were electing young John F. Kennedy, a Second World War hero who would challenge his nation to land a man on the moon within the decade, Canadians had handed a massive majority to John G. Diefenbaker, the nineteenth-century-born Prairie populist who shut down the Avro Arrow supersonic jet program. His government did, however, pass a law that extended voting rights to all First Nations people, and it enacted the Canadian Bill of Rights, precursor to the Canadian Charter of Rights and Freedoms. In Quebec, Jean Lesage was elected premier, setting the stage for the Quiet Revolution, which would shift the province out of parochialism and make it a more modern, secular society. In Western Canada, Saskatchewan was still two years away from bringing in socialized health care, which would set the standard for the eventual national model.

It was a different world, too. Nikita Khrushchev occupied the Kremlin and, claiming that history was on the Soviet Union's side, had threatened to 'bury' the West, ramping up the rhetoric of the Cold War. Fear of nuclear war was so pervasive that many countries were building secret subterranean fallout shelters to house top political and military personnel should 'the bomb' or 'the big one' be dropped. Canada was anything but immune; work had begun on the Diefenbunker near Ottawa in 1959. Meanwhile, tens of thousands of North American families were constructing their own shelters in the basements and backyards of their suburban homes.

Despite the tension of the times, it was a simpler world – or at least it seemed so on the surface. Canadians, then as now, were passionate about hockey. But it was a six-team league that they followed, not the thirty-franchise National Hockey League of today. Maurice 'The Rocket' Richard retired that year, a few months after helping his Montreal Canadiens defeat the Toronto Maple Leafs to win a fifth straight Stanley Cup. 'It was not an easy decision to make,' he told reporters, 'but I guess I finally realized this week that the game is getting too fast for me.'[3]

In fact, the sports world would never be quite the same again after 1960, when a brash young fighter named Cassius Clay won gold at the Rome Olympics, then began a professional career that would see him dominate heavyweight boxing, change his name to Muhammad Ali, and become the prototype for the outspoken superstar athlete.

Elvis Presley, returning from his army stint, resumed his rule over the radio airwaves with two of his biggest hits: 'It's Now or Never' and 'Are You Lonesome To-night?' He shared the top of the charts with a dance craze song – Chubby Checker's 'The Twist.' The Beatles had yet to make an appearance on the Top Forty pop music charts. They were still learning their rock 'n' roll craft at the Indra Club and the Kaiserkeller in Hamburg and were two years away from releasing 'Love Me Do.'

This was a time before multiplex theatres, when moviegoers flocked to auditorium-like movie houses to watch Marilyn Monroe and Yves Montand in *Let's Make Love* and Clark Gable and Sophia Loren in *It Started in Naples*. The previous year's Best Picture, *Ben-Hur*, was still playing (films didn't go to video or DVD back then), and Alfred Hitchcock's *Psycho* was scaring people out of taking showers. Jack Lemmon, a pixyish Shirley MacLaine, and Fred MacMurray were scandalizing audiences in *The Apartment*, a film that would go on to win the Best Picture Oscar. Sean Connery was two years away from introducing himself as 'Bond ... James Bond.' Steve McQueen had not yet attempted *The Great Escape*, and Stanley Kubrick was eight years away from unveiling *2001: A Space Odyssey*.

At home, people were watching *The Twilight Zone* and *Hawaiian Eye* on their black-and-white televisions. This was a pre–reality-show TV world in which wholesome family fare like *My Three Sons* and *The Andy Griffith Show* were beginning long runs. In Britain, 1960 audiences were about to discover *Coronation Street*, which debuted in December of that year and is still going strong.

In literature, everyone was reading Harper Lee's novel, *To Kill a Mockingbird*. Published in July 1960, it would go on to win the Pulitzer Prize. Walter M. Miller, Jr, painted a word portrait of life after nuclear holocaust with *A Canticle for Liebowitz*. Closer to home, Farley Mowat had begun his Top of the World trilogy with *Ordeal by Ice*. Margaret Atwood had yet to graduate from the University of Toronto, and her first novel, *The Edible Woman*, would not be published for another nine years.

The world in which Till and McCulloch made their discovery was one in which the Barbie doll was still a new toy. A world without Rocky Balboa, Don Corleone, or Captain Kirk. There were no Rolling Stones. It was a world in which the Austin Motor Company was selling $1,295 cars at 250 dealerships across Canada. It was before Martin Luther King, Jr, won the Nobel Peace Prize. New York City's World Trade Center had not yet been built. IBM – whose chairman Thomas Watson had once predicted a world market 'for maybe five computers' – was preparing to introduce its new Selectric typewriter. In this world there was no Internet, no cellphones, and no text messaging.

It was a world in which the existence of stem cells – the fundamental units required for organs and tissue and blood and bone – was still an hypothesis.

Awe and Dread

To borrow from Dickens, the era during which James Till and Ernest McCulloch were working away in their OCI labs on Sherbourne Street in the early 1960s truly was the best of times and the worst of times for scientific research.

In a *Globe and Mail* article published on the first day of 1960, staff writer David Spurgeon looked toward the coming decade and declared that 'the science fiction of the early Fifties will become the fact of the Sixties.' How could it not? 'Man's achievements in satellite and rocket technology alone during the past decade have constituted an advance never before approached in terms of scientific techniques.'[4]

Just across the page, his colleague George Bain was less effusive about achievements of the decade just ended, which he suggested might become known as the 'Fretful Fifties.' But he did offer some optimism that the Big Four summit (the United States, the Soviet Union, the United Kingdom, and France) that was due to begin in Paris in the spring might mark the beginning of meaningful negotiations on nuclear disarmament.[5] Bain's hopefulness, it turned out, was misplaced. The capture of an American U-2 spy plane over Soviet airspace two weeks before the talks led to their early collapse and sent the message around the world that the Cold War was not about to thaw any time soon and indeed had grown several degrees colder.

Governments around the world were investing heavily in science, but there were fears about nuclear technology. Aside from its use in weapons production, nuclear energy was being developed in the postwar period as a new way to generate electric power and to make isotopes for medical use. But it was capable of causing catastrophic damage. It had already unleashed the new man-made disease of 'radiation sickness.' In 1952, one of the world's first major nuclear reactor accidents occurred on Canadian soil. The NRX reactor at Chalk River, Ontario, suffered a partial meltdown, spewing radioactive material at the site and intensifying atomic angst across North America.

Understandably, then, the subject of science in the early 1960s often provoked two conflicting responses, sometimes from the same person at the same time. One was an undeniable sense of awe that science was going to make it possible to walk on the moon and send spacecraft to other planets to solve the riddles of the universe. The other was an overriding sense of dread, that scientific advances were pushing humanity ever closer to extinction.

Only fifteen years earlier, the United States had hastened the end of the Second World War and launched the Atomic Age by dropping nuclear bombs on Hiroshima and Nagasaki, killing somewhere between 150,000 and 246,000 Japanese. The Soviet Union then accelerated the nuclear arms race, testing its first nuclear weapon in 1949.

The 1950s had been a decade of exhilarating achievement, especially in health research. Many of the standard medical procedures we take for granted today were discovered or developed during those years, which receive more attention for the public's fascination with the hula hoop and the birth of rock 'n' roll than for the eradication of polio and the discovery of DNA.

Jonas Salk's vaccine was proven safe and effective in 1955, easing the pervasive fear of a disease that killed or disabled thousands of people, most of them children, when it raged across continents every summer. Polio, the Salk Institute declares, was 'the most frightening scourge of the time.'[6] The vaccines developed by Salk and Albert Sabin provided peace of mind to millions of parents. While polio still exists in a handful of developing countries, it has largely been eradicated.

The 'secret to life itself'[7] was revealed in 1953 when Britain's James Watson and Francis Crick, with a little help from Maurice Wilkins, came up with the double-helix model for DNA, the molecule responsible for transferring traits from generation to generation. The trio won the 1962 Nobel Prize in Physiology and Medicine for their discovery.

As the *Globe and Mail* turn-of-the-decade article illustrates, the 1950s also saw developments in heart surgery to treat disease and correct congenital defects, better understanding of the biochemical basis of mental illnesses, and improvements in fighting infection with antibiotics. But there was still a stealthy killer out there: cancer, a truly democratic disease that, then as now, does not discriminate between the young and the old, the rich and the poor.

Ernest McCulloch, who dedicated much of his life to finding a cure for leukemia, provided one of the most eloquent descriptions of the insidious nature of cancer:

> The disease begins as a genetic change in a single cell. The cell becomes less responsive to normal mechanisms that restrain growth. The result is a population derived from a single cell (a clonal population), all of whose members carry the genetic change that began the process. The clone may remain localized long enough to grow into a recognizable tumour, but invasion of adjacent tissues usually occurs. Early or late in its history the cancerous clone gains access to the blood system; cells then migrate to distant organs, where cells initiate new subclones, called metastases. Some tumours, particularly those of the blood and lymph systems, are almost always widely spread when the disease is sufficiently advanced to allow for diagnosis. As long as the malignant clone remains localized, it can be removed surgically or the growth capacity of the cancer cells can be destroyed by radiation. When the tumour has spread, systemic treatment is needed, usually with chemotherapeutic drugs.[8]

The OCI, where Till and McCulloch worked, had been founded to treat cancer patients in a centralized location; equipment-intensive radiation therapy could be administered safely in the clinics while researchers worked in their labs to unlock the secrets of the disease.

Radiation therapy was nothing new. In the early 1900s, Marie Curie, who coined the term 'radioactivity,' won two Nobel Prizes for her pioneering work in radiation and her discovery of the elements radium and polonium. She was an innovator in the use of radioactive isotopes to treat cancer. Up until the mid-century, physicians were using radiation to combat cancer cells by giving patients heavy-duty X-ray treatments or implanting radium near their tumours. These treatments, however, were expensive, difficult to administer, and limited in their effectiveness.

Things changed significantly after scientists at the Chalk River nuclear facility created a better, cheaper source of radiation in the form of the Cobalt-60 isotope. The University of Saskatchewan's Harold Johns, who would go on to be Till's boss in the Physics Division of the OCI, was instrumental in designing the Cobalt-60 therapy unit, where gamma rays were beamed at cancer tumours to inflict damage on the cells' DNA. Introduced in the early 1950s in Saskatchewan and Ontario, the treatment became widely known as the 'Cobalt bomb,' a label that some attributed to the awesome apparatus required to deliver the beam – although a CBC Radio report compared one to 'a small-sized cement mixer.'[9] Others interpreted the title as a nod to a non-destructive use of nuclear technology.[10] Regardless, it dramatically improved cure rates for cervical cancer and for deep-set tumours in the bladder and lung.[11,12]

In the late 1940s, Leon O. Jacobson of the University of Chicago had begun pioneering research into radiation therapy based largely on what he had learned from his time as a physician on the Manhattan Project, working with the team that built the atom bomb during the Second World War.

Jacobson studied the effects of radiation on the body's ability to make blood, a process called hematopoiesis. He zapped mice with massive doses of radiation in a crude arrangement in which their spleens were protected with lead shields. After about a week, the spleen-shielded mice were still alive and blood formation was revived in their bone marrow.

As Alison Kraft explains in her 2009 paper, 'Manhattan Transfer: Lethal Radiation, Bone Marrow Transplantation, and the Birth of Stem Cell Biology, ca. 1942–1961,' the work that Jacobson and his colleague Egon Lorenz were engaged in was originally aimed not at treating cancer but at studying the effects of radiation and finding ways to reverse them. (Till and McCulloch were also on the case: research they were doing in the late 1950s and early 1960s was funded in part by grants from

Canada's Defence Research Board.) Lorenz, Kraft explains, took Jacobson's idea further when he injected irradiated mice with clean bone marrow and found that they recovered.

The great hope was that a drug could be developed to combat radiation sickness after exposure to radiation from an enemy attack or nuclear generator meltdown. While such a cure was never found, the research proved particularly applicable to treating leukemia – cancer of the blood – and spurred scientists to investigate bone marrow transplantation as a treatment. According to Kraft,

> BMT (bone marrow transplantation) was not developed by clinicians for the treatment of cancer. Rather, building on research undertaken during the Manhattan Project, it was developed first as a research tool by a group of specialists investigating the biological effects of lethal radiation and seeking a means for its treatment. In the course of this research it became apparent that within the bone marrow there was an 'active principle,' the means to regenerate the blood system.[13]

Bone marrow transplantation as a leukemia therapy was in its early experimental stages in the late 1950s. E. Donnall Thomas reported in 1957 that he had carried out the first human bone marrow transplants on six terminally ill patients. He went on to win the Nobel Prize in 1990 for his work as the driving force of bone marrow transplantation. The treatment he developed is common practice today and saves lives in hospitals around the world. In 1960, however, a diagnosis of leukemia was almost certainly a death sentence.

Naturally, then, along with the Cold War and fears about radiation, the public was increasingly anxious about cancer. While treatments like the Cobalt bomb had improved the odds for survival, the disease was still taking lives at an alarming rate. Besides investing in fallout shelters, governments were making cancer research and treatment a major priority.

It was this sense of urgency that led to the creation of the OCI and the inclusion of researchers at the Sherbourne Street site. A much-told story has it that Ontario Premier Leslie Frost shrugged at plans for what was to be a five-storey cancer treatment centre and ordered two floors be added, purely for research. His abrupt decision launched a pioneering cancer research centre where Till and McCulloch would be brought together.

3

The Impossible Partnership

The boxes are stuffed with folder after folder of hand-drawn charts and graphs that plot the results of long-ago experiments. There are old carbon copy sheets of carefully typed letters and pages with nothing but columns of figures recording now forgotten calculations, many written carefully in pencil with the occasional erasure and correction. It is an impressive collection: the lab notes, correspondence, and collected works of James Till and Ernest McCulloch take up almost eighty-five feet of shelf space – the equivalent of six average-sized automobiles parked in a line – in the University of Toronto Archives. There is, however, not a single scrap or scribble remaining from the prep work they did for their crucial 1961 *Radiation Research* paper that proved the existence of stem cells. Till thinks it was all discarded early on. The pair only started keeping more organized records after that initial breakthrough, he says, apologetically. 'At the time, you don't think you're going to be doing anything historic.'

McCulloch, whose last few years were wracked with illnesses and hospital stays, died in January 2011. An infection had cost him an eye two years before his death. In the last few months of his life, walking was difficult and he tired easily, but he remained mentally sharp and still read voraciously, a lifelong habit that became his principal enjoyment. That said, the man with the once dazzling ability to recite whole passages of Shakespeare or to retrieve a particularly relevant paper from a teetering tower of reports on his cluttered desk sometimes struggled to remember the name of a particular Canadian author he admired.

As in his younger days, though, he did not suffer fools lightly; he was quick to point out passages of his book about the Ontario Cancer Institute that would answer specific questions. 'Have you read my book?' he would ask. He was just as quick to offer praise and to direct attention to former colleagues, pointing out their work and essential contributions. Having taken stock of his professional life by writing *The Ontario Cancer Institute: Successes and Reverses at Sherbourne Street* (McGill-Queen's University Press, 2003), he did not appear to harbour grudges or nurse slights. Knowing that he was nearing the end of his life, he had no scores to settle.

Till is an old man now, but he retains a certain spryness. Born five years after McCulloch, he stays trim and fit by curling throughout the winter. He stands tall, if a little stiffly, and laughs easily, often at himself. He has a firm handshake and gimlet eyes that one long-time colleague describes as producing 'a beam that is so concentrated on you, it's almost as if he's reassuring himself that what you're saying is credible and correct.' Not given to hyperbole, he favours precision. While he will give you his honest assessment of the subject at hand, if it isn't an area of his interest or expertise, he'll simply say, 'I wouldn't know' or 'I have no documentation.' He deflects praise or redirects it to those he thinks deserve it more. But he is not without pride. He refers to the work he did with McCulloch as 'one of the few things that stood the test of time' in the controversial field of stem cell science.

He also has some regrets. He speaks candidly about how a life dedicated to science kept him from spending time with his wife Joyce and their three children. Along with the travel to conferences, he put in very long hours at the OCI. 'It wasn't just fiddling with test tubes,' he says. 'I had other collaborations going on, so I participated in a lot of other people's projects. And there was grant writing and committee work. I could tolerate it a lot more than Ernest. It all added up.'

McCulloch could not recall their first encounter. Neither does Till, but he does remember one particular event in, he thinks, 1958 during their early days at the OCI. 'The research program started with two divisions: Physics Division and Biological Research. Arthur Ham, who was the first head of the Biological Research Division, thought people should get to know each other. He didn't like to go out, so he organized meetings at his house in Don Mills. I remember meeting several times in the basement of his house. I remember Ernest McCulloch giving a talk, quite informally, about his interests and I thought, "This is interesting!"'

McCulloch recalled that it was Harold Johns, a pioneer in the delivery of cancer radiation therapy and a major influence on Till's academic and professional life, who brought them together. 'I wanted to irradiate mice and inject them with bone marrow as part of my experimental program. Harold had a rule that nobody could use radiation in that building without a physicist. Harold's reputation was built on accurate measurements of radiation; he wasn't going to have any damn biologist ruining his reputation by misusing his machines. Jim volunteered to be the radiation expert and keep me on the straight and narrow. As soon as we got together, we found we worked well together.'

Different Paths

That the two men could even stand each other let alone work closely together for more than two decades came as a surprise to many. 'It was an impossible partnership,' says Lou Siminovitch, an early colleague who went on to become one of Canada's pioneers in genetics. 'They're so different. Ernest could quote poetry, he read enormously. He was a highly emotional person and full of ideas. He was one of the most imaginative people I ever worked with. Jim was a farmer … he was rough-hewn. He was very pragmatic, down to earth. He was very clever, very analytical, very rigorous.'

Victor Ling, a Till recruit at OCI whose discovery of p-glycoprotein advanced the understanding of multi-drug resistance in cancer therapies, says that McCulloch was creative, intuitive, and passionate about his work. 'I think he dreamed about what the outcome might be, even before other people could recognize it. Jim Till is also very eloquent, but he's much more quantitative, having a physicist's approach to understanding any data that were generated. He'd analyse it, put it into a mathematical formula if possible.'

The life paths that led the two men to the OCI could not have been more different. One came from a wealthy Ontario family. The other was the son of a Prairie homesteader.

Ernest Armstrong 'Bun' McCulloch was born in Toronto on 27 April 1926. Armstrong was his mother's maiden name. 'Bun' is a gift he was given as an infant that he tried unsuccessfully to lose for the rest of his life. 'It was given to me in my cradle. My grandmother called me Bun. At that time, nicknames were the fad. My mother had a nickname: she was called Tad. She had a twin sister who was called Jim. Her older sister was called Blue. My older sister got called Tot. It was common in those days for everybody to have some sort of a peculiar name.'

For what it's worth, Till does not refer to his long-time partner as Bun. He is one of the very few who call him Ernest, and in correspondence, he uses 'EAM.' Almost everyone else who has ever worked with McCulloch refers to him as Bun. Women colleagues take it a step further – to them, he is 'Bunny.'

'I can't shake it,' said McCulloch. 'People that I meet, I'd give my proper name to and for years they use my proper name. And then they run into somebody from Toronto and it all gets lost.'

James Edgar Till was born on the Saskatchewan side of the provincial border town of Lloydminster on 25 August 1931, in the depths of the Great Depression. The son of a pioneer who had come to Canada from England to homestead, Till remembers a boyhood spent helping out on the family's Alberta farm. Those were the days before combines came into common use, when harvesting wheat meant cutting the stalks into sheaves, then bundling them up in stooks for the thresher.

'We worked from five in the morning until nine in the night. We had one quarter section that was all one field, all planted to wheat. It was cut and my job was to stook it. I remember looking at one hundred and sixty acres of sheaves and thinking, "I've got to stand all those on end!" But you just do it. You just lean in and do it.'

Till, though, didn't just lean in and do it. Instead of letting his mind wander while his body did the monotonous labour, he would run time-and-motion studies 'to make myself more efficient.' He did the same when it came time to place the stooks on a bundle rack to be hauled to the thresher. 'I wasn't strong enough to do what the other people were doing. They had four-pronged forks that we called straw forks and they would just toss those stooks onto the bundle rack with one sweeping motion. I couldn't do that, I was a teenager and I wasn't strong enough. So again I had to do time-and-motion studies on myself to keep it efficient, and even then I couldn't quite keep up.'

A farmboy with a head for figures, Till remembers life getting easier when combines came along. He recalls their arrival clearly. 'When we got our first combine there was some kind of rail strike going on and they couldn't deliver it past North Battleford. There were three combines to be picked up and a group of us, I represented my family, went to North Battleford, got these combines, put them together, and drove them to Lloydminster, one hundred miles away, at five miles an hour. I got to know the scenery pretty well along the way.'

For Till, the family farm back in Alberta was always an ace in the hole should his research career fall through. Even while he was making stem cell history in the early 1960s, he was still going back to the farm for a week or two every fall to help bring in the harvest. Knowing that the farm was there meant he never had to worry about taking on difficult research challenges, he says. If all else failed, if the experiments proved to be all for naught, he knew he could always go back to growing wheat.

McCulloch, by contrast, was a child of privilege. His father was a doctor, as were two uncles. He grew up on Warren Road south of St Clair Avenue. His family owned a cottage at Ahmic Lake north of Toronto, and he learned how to sail in the summers. He was educated at Upper Canada College, where Ontario's elite has always sent its boys to become young gentlemen and men of business. Sailing aside, McCulloch was dismal at sports and didn't fit in with the upper-crust school's sporting crowd. 'I'm ham-handed in every possible way.' He even disliked the great Canadian pastime: 'Hockey is just a bunch of guys running around on skates, as far as I can see. I just find it dull.'

McCulloch was of Scottish ancestry. 'Any time I refuse to spend money I always blame it on my ancestors, but I've never actually been to Scotland.' He remembered the Toronto of his youth as 'a mean, nasty, and miserable little town. It was narrow-minded. If you've read Mordecai Richler's *Oh Canada! Oh Quebec!* everything he said about Montreal – because it was nasty – you could say about Toronto. I was brought up with a strong anti-Semitic bias, but you only have to meet a number of Jewish people to get rid of that in a hurry.

'There was only one place where there was live theatre – the Royal Alex – and it was only open some of the time. [Toronto] was a miserable place and what saved it, of course, was when the immigrants arrived, principally Italians. There was no place outside of two or three restaurants where you could get [even] a mediocre meal as I grew up. The Italians came in, everybody came in, and now you can get any kind of food that you like. And I've always thought that we had an unwritten sort of pact, which is that if you come to Toronto, you start your restaurants and preserve your culture – but the rule is that you have to share it. Toronto is much, much better now.'

A conversation with McCulloch could go anywhere. He was as comfortable discussing Edward Gibbon's *The Decline and Fall of the Roman Empire* ('If you want a liberal education, read Gibbon') or Robert Montgomery's 1941 vehicle *Here Comes Mr. Jordan* ('A marvellous movie!') as he was parsing the intricacies of blood cell regeneration.

Till, in stark contrast, thinks in straighter lines and speaks more cautiously, though he can get animated about the investigation he and other OCI colleagues conducted in 1967 to assess the impact of sweeping on the trajectory of a curling stone. (He later wrote in an article, published by the Royal Society of Canada, about how sweeping can turn 'a well-thrown stone into a superbly thrown one.')

If Till's relentless attention to detail came naturally, his sense of the importance of getting things right in the science lab was honed while working on his master's degree in the early 1950s with Harold Johns at the University of Saskatchewan in Saskatoon. Till went there for his undergrad degree after the school offered him a small scholarship. With no money in his family tree, every dollar mattered to a young Jim Till.

Johns, who had pioneered the Cobalt bomb radiation treatment, was Till's mentor long before the term came into vogue. 'He was my adviser. He was unique ... He had a great talent and he actually never grew up. He had the curiosity and enthusiasm of a teenager all his life, which is a remarkable thing. That's a rigorous mind, I mean. He didn't put up with anything second-rate. He was competitive. They used to say that he would make anything, including tiddlywinks, into a bloody contact sport.'

Clearly, Till did not choose an easy guru. Siminovitch, in *Reflections on a Life in Science*, describes Johns as 'almost ruthless with those who did not measure up, especially those who did not demonstrate a proper work ethic.' The tough-minded, results-oriented Johns would prove to be instrumental in Till's career both at school and later on, when the two later reconnected at the OCI.

'While I was in Saskatoon,' Till says, 'I decided I wanted to get more involved in biological research, because I thought the radiation physics side of it didn't leave a lot of room to manoeuvre and the important unresolved problems, in terms of radiation effects, were on the biological side. Harold had something to do with that. He suggested we look into that. So I went for a biophysics program and that's how I ended up at Yale.'

Till was able to earn a spot at the Ivy League school in 1954 thanks to a fellowship from the National Cancer Institute of Canada. While in Saskatoon, he had become friends with fellow Johns acolyte Gordon Whitmore. 'In fact, it was Gordon that recruited me into research in the first place, it wasn't Harold himself. He and I both went to Yale to the Biophysics Department. We made a sort of suicide pact that we would both try this out and support each other.'

The suicide pact proved unnecessary. Both men succeeded in their studies at one of the top institutions of learning in the world. PhD in hand, Till declined an offer to stay on. 'They offered me an assistant professorship at Yale in the department, but I didn't want to stay in the United States. I was looking for jobs in Canada and I could only find one in the biophysics area, which is my degree. There was a lab at [the] National Research Council in Ottawa, I had an offer to go there. Then Harold Johns offered me an option with the new OCI when it was finished in Toronto.

'I don't remember the exact sequence but they offered this deal that I could have a postdoctoral year working with Lou Siminovitch. I knew he had made some major contributions to microbiology when he worked at the Pasteur Institute in Paris. They worked out some kind of deal where if I went to Connaught Laboratories with Lou and his research colleague Angus Graham, the OCI would pay for it.'

It would be a pleasant setting. The Connaught Laboratories were located out on Steeles Avenue, on former farmland that had been donated to the University of Toronto. 'Harold was interested in me coming to join his new Physics Division staff at the OCI, so it would be a good way to keep me around for a year until the new building opened. I thought, "That's terrific; that's the best deal I'll get."'

So, in 1957, Till said no to Yale and came back to Canada.

McCulloch had dutifully followed the family career path to become a doctor, earning his medical degree at the University of Toronto in 1948. A brilliant student, he earned the opportunity to study in London, England – an experience that began to change his mind about what he wanted to do with his life. 'I was at the Lister Institute, learning to do research. I wasn't really doing research, I was experiencing research. They showed me that research could be a very pleasant occupation. It was interesting.'

He returned to Canada in 1949 and interned at the Toronto General Hospital until 1952. He then became an assistant resident at Sunnybrook Hospital through 1953, according to the biographical note prepared by the University of Toronto Archives for the Ernest Armstrong McCulloch Fonds. But he kept a foot in the laboratory as a research fellow in pathology at the Banting Institute. He co-authored a paper titled 'The Response of the Renal Circulation of the Rabbit to Adrenaline,' published in the *British Journal of Surgery* in 1952, and began building up his expertise in hematology. 'I was trained as a doctor. I completed all postgraduate requirements and I was a specialist in internal medicine. So I had a lot of medical training.'

In 1954, McCulloch joined the University of Toronto's Department of Medicine as a teacher but continued to see patients on the wards of the Toronto General Hospital. His patient load, however, dwindled over the years because he wasn't devoting the time required to build up a roster of them. 'I continued to teach medicine and gave lectures on hematology,' he said during a bedside interview a few months before his death. 'But I had fewer and fewer patients. If you want to have a lot of patients, you have to run a practice. A medical practice is a business and I have never had a head for business.'

When McCulloch was offered the position of Head of Hematology in the Biology Division of the OCI in 1957, he snapped it up. The shift soon brought an end to his private practice. 'I couldn't do both patient work and research. If you had patient responsibilities, you were always interrupted. After a while, I gave it up.'

His decision to become a salaried researcher did not sit well with some members of his family, particularly his older sister, who was disappointed in him. 'You see, I had all these advantages. I went to Upper Canada College. I got a medical education … With all those advantages I could have made a lot of money. But I didn't. It shows that everybody has their criteria for success. Mine wasn't money. I've always been reasonably well paid. I'm not complaining about poverty. But [scientists] are not paid the way a practising physician would be paid. In other words, if I'd followed the family business and gone into practice I would have had lots of money and a big house in Rosedale, not a little house.'

His sister's disappointment notwithstanding, McCulloch was born to be a research scientist. The scientific method – observing, questioning, hypothesizing, experimenting, weighing results, drawing conclusions – may well have been encoded in his DNA. Abandoning his first career had been a difficult choice, but it led him to a place where he was clearly destined to succeed.

'He was not really trained as a scientist,' says Siminovitch. 'It wasn't just that he didn't have a PhD; he wasn't trained. He learned very quickly.'

Till recalls that McCulloch was sensitive about not having a doctorate. 'I remember [him] once saying, "You should be the supervisor for Andy [Becker, who would go on to play a pivotal role in their work] because I haven't had that much experience with academic programs." Which was true, because he did not have a PhD, he had not been through a PhD program himself, although he'd done postgraduate research in England. He didn't talk about it much, but I think he was rather sensitive about it himself, that he hadn't had the proper academic apprenticeship.'

For his part, McCulloch referred to his medical degree as 'my only authority, the only degree I have.' He also rejected the stereotype that a scientist was someone who bent over a microscope or poked at Petri dishes all day, oblivious to life beyond the laboratory. He did not believe in types. 'Scientists are all individuals. You can't lump us together and say, "This is what a scientist is." They talk about artistic communities and how vibrant they are and so on. But it's nothing at all compared to research.'

If McCulloch strayed outside the family tradition in his choice of career, he also did so in his choice of a bride, marrying Ona, a New Zealander who worked as a nurse at Sunnybrook Hospital, instead of some Old Money matron-in-waiting. Together they had five children. 'That would now be considered sinful,' he said, 'but when we were having children, five was not unusual.' They raised them in their 'little' house in Rosedale.

According to a tribute to McCulloch published in the *Globe and Mail*, he courted his wife Ona with verses of Tennyson's *Ulysses*. His son Jim said that the romance between his parents was 'like crazy ... it was a storybook.' He recalled his father reading Charles Dickens's *A Christmas Carol* every December. J.R.R. Tolkien's *Lord of the Rings* trilogy and *The Hobbit* were also favourites for reading aloud to the children.[14]

While his wife was a believer, McCulloch did not have much use for religion. 'My wife is Catholic. I'm not religious. If you do science, one can't imagine a god that has narrow views. It's hard to imagine a god that ... what's the proper word? ... thinks that this is right and that's wrong.'

Early Days at the OCI

Till and McCulloch were recruited to the team of bright young cancer researchers that was being assembled at the OCI labs atop the Princess Margaret Hospital. As the newly created Department of Medical Biophysics,[15] the operation was part of the University of Toronto; but its off-campus location, with all the scientists gathered under one roof instead of scattered around different buildings, gave it something of a pirate ship appeal. Its Sherbourne Street location must have solidified the sense that it was separate from ivy-clad academia: the avenue of once stately homes occupied by Toronto's upper crust had become a strip of seedy rooming houses with a clientele of street people, drug addicts, and prostitutes.

McCulloch maintained that the isolation was 'the best thing that ever happened to us – there was no one looking over our shoulders.' Not only was the new institution physically separate, but its early leadership was determined that it would stand apart. The goal was not to be the best cancer research facility in Canada – it was to take on the world. Certainly the OCI had the leadership to do it. Johns, after his success in Saskatchewan in developing the Cobalt bomb, was an internationally respected innovator in the delivery of radiation for cancer treatment. As such, he was the perfect person to head the Physics Division. In Arthur Ham, the Biological Research Division had a man who had literally written the book on microscopic anatomy. His *Histology* textbook would become required reading for several generations of medical students.

'Johns and Ham insisted that we were internationalists,' said McCulloch. 'What your work was judged against was the international standard. We didn't go to Canadian meetings – we went to American meetings to present our stuff. We were able to develop what I insist on calling a culture. You had to be able to explain what you were doing. Because it was biophysics. If you were a biologist you had to explain what you were doing to a physicist and if you were a physicist you had to explain what you were doing to a biologist. We all became quite good a giving public presentations.'

The roster of the OCI's early recruits – unproven, raw talents with a smattering of established hands – now reads like a Who's Who of Canadian medical research. Along with Till, the Physics Division included Gordon Whitmore, who had returned to Canada from Yale with Till and eventually would succeed Ham and Johns as head of the Medical Biophysics Department.[16] Robert Bruce, another Johns acolyte, who had a medical degree as well as a PhD in physics, was an early proponent of computerized medical records and did ground-breaking work in cancer chemotherapy. He has devoted much of his career to the impact of diet and nutrition on colon cancer. On the biology side, there was Siminovitch, who would go on to create what became the University of Toronto's Department of Medical Genetics and to found the Samuel Lunenfeld Research Institute at Mount Sinai Hospital. Bernhard Cinader is credited with pioneering the study of immunology in Canada. Clarence Fuerst led investigations into bacterial viruses. And there was Rose Sheinin, an early promoter of the link between viruses and cancer as well as a tireless advocate for women's equality in science and academia.

They did not operate like members of a university department. As Siminovitch explains in *Reflections*, the OCI's basic scientists were not offered academic tenure and 'understood that their future security lay in their success in research and, to some extent, their contribution to the Institute.' The scientists' salaries did not even come from the university; instead, they were pass-through funds from the Ontario Cancer Treatment and Research Foundation. The scientists were also encouraged to seek funding from other sources, such as the Medical Research Council (forerunner to the Canadian Institutes of Health Research), the National Cancer Institute, and the U.S. National Institutes of Health. From the earliest days, the pressure was on to do outstanding work.

The OCI leadership was far in front of the pack in encouraging 'bonding' between the scientists. Long before outdoor team-building exercises became trendy, the scientists were abandoning their labs on Sherbourne Street to take part in annual three-day retreats at rustic cottages owned by Johns and his family at Boshkung Lake in Ontario's Haliburton County. Between water skiing, hikes in the woods, and campfire sessions, the scientists presented their latest theories and discussed where they hoped to take their work. It was recreational, but hardly fun and games.

'We would sit on a big rock with a big blackboard and each person would describe what they were doing with their work and where they were going,' recalls Bruce. 'Then there was a general free-for-all. You could be criticized at any time throughout it. The hard part was a lot of people didn't quite come up to standards and got turfed out. There were people who suffered in that situation. It was fun for the people who survived, but I'm sure it wasn't fun for a lot of people.'

In his book, Siminovitch concurs that the OCI could be a crucible for some: 'I also learned some important lessons, such as that no matter how good a place may be, it is not necessarily the right environment for everyone. I witnessed three breakdowns in my office during my tenure. "Professional" biochemists found it inhospitable.'[17]

McCulloch could be devastating in his criticism of those he felt had missed the mark, once telling a visiting postdoctoral fellow who had just made a presentation at the OCI to 'burn all your slides!'

For Bob Phillips, an early recruit from the United States who would go on to be a major player in Canadian cancer research, the OCI was a great place to be a young scientist. 'I think none of us realized how unique a place it was at that time,' he says. 'Lou Siminovitch and Harold Johns believed in essentially two critical things. There had to be excellence – they just did not compromise on excellence. We were competing on the international scene, so we had to be working on research that was the best of the best. Second, the only way you can do that is to be totally open and interactive. So the people would always interact, with discussions between groups. And it was very stimulating. You get a lot of good ideas by talking to the physicists and talking to the clinicians. Other places didn't have the same degree of interaction. People were high achievers, but I didn't detect jealousy. If somebody succeeded, then everybody celebrated the success. If you won a prize I'd say, "Great! Let's go out and have a beer." I wouldn't say, "Oh, that jerk."'

In this tough, challenging, and often exhilarating environment, Till and McCulloch set about their work.

'Jim and Bun joined forces early on,' says OCI alumnus Mike McBurney, who is Program Director of Cancer Therapeutics at the Ottawa Health Research Institute. 'They are quite different people. Bun was always the dreamer and Jim was the guy who figured out how to do it. It worked out extremely well.'

Into the Mystery

Scientific researchers have egos. It's part of what drives them to be first to find something out – so that their names and their institutions will forever be linked with a discovery or innovation. Till and McCulloch were no different in this regard. They both embraced the OCI 'let's take on the world' philosophy. It gave them the nerve to search for one of the most puzzling pieces in biology: the stem cell.

If the biggest mystery in biology is the source of life – as in, what drives a sperm cell to swim to the egg so that together they create a zygote? – then the next-biggest question is: How does a body build and maintain itself? The stem cell is the still not fully understood answer to that question. It is the body's most basic building block. It is the original cellular unit that can transform itself into other units that (in the womb) create blood and bone, heart and lung, eyes and ears, and (throughout a lifespan) make repairs to or replace worn or broken parts.

But stem cells don't simply transform themselves into other cells (a process called differentiation) to build what the body needs and then, their work done, quietly disappear. They are more than progenitors of other cells. They also replicate themselves – in an unrefined, undifferentiated state – so that they can stick around to answer the call later when the blood system needs rebuilding after it has been ravaged by leukemia, or the kidneys need repair after they've been struck and damaged. It's this ability to create new versions of itself (self-renewal) that sets the stem cell apart, that is its key characteristic.

But at what point in the differentiation process does a stem cell stop being a stem cell? Are there degrees of 'stem-cellness'? Totipotent stem cells in the embryo can produce anything the body requires. Then it's a sliding scale from pluripotent to multipotent to, essentially, one-trick pony adult stem cells. Bone marrow stem cells, for example, specialize in producing bone marrow for making blood; neural stem cells make neurons. And what if you could manipulate already differentiated stem cells that do one thing – such as those that line the intestines – so that they did something altogether different – such as producing insulin for the pancreas? That ability to take on a new assignment is called plasticity. What would you call those stem cells?

The very existence of stem cells was still open to debate when McCulloch walked into his lab on that Sunday in 1960 and made his discovery. Unlike today's technological world, in which advances in electron microscopes have given scientists the wherewithal to capture and colorize images of stem cells growing on the walls of supporting cells of connective tissue called fibroblasts, back then the idea of stem cells was exactly that – an idea. An hypothesis. A theory.

It was, however, a theory with considerable history behind it, thanks to the convergence of Industrial Age tools with natural human curiosity. The development of microscopes in the 1800s made it possible for scientists to take a good look at the basic unit of life – the cell – and to ponder its origins, forms, and functions.

In 1868, a brilliant German man of letters named Ernst Haeckel, an early adopter of Darwin's theory of natural selection and the evolution of complex creatures from simpler stock, theorized that all multicelled organisms has a single-celled starting point – in German, a *stammzelle.* According to a commentary by Miguel Ramalho-Santos and Holger Willenbring published in the 2007 inaugural issue of the journal *Cell Stem Cell*, Haeckel also suggested that a fertilized egg in embryo could be called a stem cell.[18] That commentary explains that in 1892, German biologist Theodor Boveri pushed the definition further by proposing that cells 'along the germline lineage between the fertilized egg and committed germ cells be called stem cells.' American biologist Edmund B. Wilson has been credited with popularizing the term *stem cell;* he had used it in his 1896 book *The Cell in Development and Inheritance*.

At about the same time, again according to Ramalho-Santos and Willenbring, 'research on the development and regeneration of the hematopoietic system raised the question of whether a common precursor of the various cell types of the blood existed.' As early as 1896, they report, the term stem cell was being used to describe 'a precursor cell capable of giving rise to both red and white blood cells.' Debate over its existence continued well into the twentieth century. If a blood-forming stem cell had become something of a Holy Grail, researchers were getting closer by the mid-1950s, largely as an offshoot to the urgent search to develop anti-radiation drugs in the event of a nuclear attack or nuclear generator disaster.

The University of Chicago's Leon Jacobson had thrown the debate open with his radiation experiments on spleen-shielded mice. Their survival indicated that some kind of 'recovery factor' was at work. His colleague Egon Lorenz fortified that notion with his success in transplanting clean bone marrow into irradiated mice to bring about their recovery. However, as Alison Kraft describes in her 'Manhattan Transfer' paper, scientific opinion differed through the mid-1950s over whether it was 'a humoral factor' involving secretion of hormones that triggered mice's recovery (as Jacobson advocated) or a cell-based recovery (as a prominent group of biophysicists in Harwell, England, and others proposed). Toward the end of the decade, the latter hypothesis was proved true, though the former was not fully discarded. As Kraft explains: 'Confirmation of the cellular nature of the "recovery factor" did not preclude the possibility of hormonal involvement.'[19]

It was against this backdrop that Till and McCulloch approached their early experiments. So when McCulloch saw the bumps embedded in the mouse spleens, which seemed to correlate with the doses of marrow the animals had received, he began to think they might contain blood-forming cells – biologically speaking, they might be clones derived from a few of the transplanted cells. This seemed to check out when he drew up some graphs to test his theory and saw that for roughly every 10,000 injected marrow cells, there was one nodule.

When he showed his results to Till the next day, his partner suggested following up by directly measuring the radiation sensitivity of normal bone marrow cells; that would give a sharper and more accurate reading of what was happening. They also cut into the nodules to see what was going on in there, which confirmed McCulloch's hunch that the nodules were actually 'colonies' of blood-forming cells. Subsequent tests showed that the longer the mice were kept alive, the further along the spleen colonies were in developing what it takes to make white blood cells, red blood cells, and platelets – an amazing finding.

McCulloch and Till submitted their findings to the journal *Radiation Research* on 28 July 1960. It was published in February 1961, with a less than attention-grabbing title: 'A Direct Measurement of the Radiation Sensitivity of Normal Mouse Bone Marrow Cells.' Any journalist would criticize them for burying the lead: they didn't mention the colony-forming units until the second paragraph of the introduction, describing how 'the intravenous injection of an appropriate number of marrow cells into isologous hosts previously exposed to supralethal total-body irradiation leads to the formation of colonies of proliferating cells in the spleens of these animals.' Till got top billing only because it was his turn in the rotation – they alternated with each paper, and McCulloch had gone first in their preliminary effort with irradiated mice in 1960. From that moment on the partnership became best known as Till and McCulloch.

The paper represented an entirely new way of looking at how the body makes blood, not to mention presenting a raft of potential implications for other biological rethinks – as in, if that's true for blood, then how does the body make heart muscle, or brain tissue? But it did not immediately knock the scientific world off its axis and went largely unnoticed by the larger biology community.

'You have to remember that it was a fairly small group that was interested in this kind of work at that point,' says Till. 'This was way before all the excitement about stem cells that has happened over the last decade or so. Some experimental hematologists were interested and some radiation biologists were interested and that helped to spread it around some. But those are not mainstream fields. In terms of general interest, it didn't get much general attention until it started being quoted in textbooks.'

Till hypothesizes that because the more exciting field at the time was molecular biology – which encompasses genetics and biochemistry and focuses on the composition and roles of DNA, RNA, and proteins – work involving the ordinary cell generated far less attention. 'People were more interested in the genetic code. Cellular biology, which was what our work was about, was not in the limelight. It didn't matter what we did, the focus was on molecular biology. And rightly so: it's fascinating stuff. I would have done it myself, except I disliked chemistry.'

Another major reason for the tepid response was that the findings appeared in a publication that, though first-rate, was not a must-read for the world's biologists. 'We were studying radiation effects, so that was the logical journal for it,' says Till. 'In fact, my recollection is that the editor of *Radiation Research* had a little difficulty with the paper, that it was strange. But he was a nice guy.'

Till and McCulloch didn't hit the big time in terms of publication in prominent journals until their 1963 follow-up paper. Even then it wasn't about wanting to reach for the brass ring. 'Andy Becker wanted to see if *Nature* would publish it,' says Till. 'He was a young guy, just starting his career and, I assume, was just as concerned as most young scientists are about getting his publications into a prominent journal.'

Like McCulloch, Becker had a medical degree but was more interested in doing research than in seeing patients. That explains why he was working in the labs at the OCI as Till's PhD student instead of tending kids' tonsils or giving annual medical check-ups. After considerable trial and error – including six months of negative results – Becker adapted a method that involved using chromosomal markers created during the radiation process to trace the cells in the spleen colonies back to single cells of transplanted bone marrow. In doing so, he had found a way to prove that a single cell could produce the three types of precursors necessary to make blood.

'Karyotyping chromosomes is a painstaking technique that has a number of pitfalls,' Clelia Ganoza, Becker's wife and his spokesperson since he suffered a debilitating stroke, explained in e-mail correspondence. 'Cells can rupture during the manipulations resulting in inaccurate counts. Or the chromosomes aggregate or are too dilute to yield meaningful results. Andy, however, had an essential ingredient needed to the success of a researcher. That is the "killer" instinct, which in this context means that the goal is the important issue and the obstacles to overcome are just needed lessons towards this end. This strict perseverance is the essential ingredient to success.'

Becker was lead author (followed by McCulloch, then Till) for the 1963 *Nature* paper, 'Cytological Demonstration of the Clonal Nature of Spleen Colonies Derived from Transplanted Mouse Marrow Cells,' which proved that the colony-forming units sprang from a single cell source. It stands to this day as the definitive demonstration of the existence of stem cells.

As with the 1961 paper, however, the term 'stem cell' was not used in the *Nature* report – undoubtedly another reason why Till and McCulloch weren't attracting more mainstream attention. If their less sensational approach diminished their popular impact, the care and attention to detail that characterized all their work gave it enduring credibility. 'There weren't very many people in the world that would have taken the science to that level,' says former Till postdoc Ron Worton. 'Jim would say, "I'm sure some people think we're flogging a dead horse, but in fact as long as there's a reasonable doubt about any aspect of this stuff we're doing, it's our obligation to nail it down and prove it." You could see how that combination of Till and his rigour and McCulloch and his wild ideas complemented one another beautifully and made them the success they were.'

Till and McCulloch published a second paper in 1963, bringing Siminovitch onto the team. They studied variations in the composition of the cells in the spleen colonies, and in that way demonstrated that the colony-forming cells could give rise to new colony-forming units – an indicator of the self-renewal capacity that is crucial to the definition of a stem cell. Siminovitch, who had worked with Nobel laureates at the Pasteur Institute in Paris, initiated the project and was lead author on the paper, 'The Distribution of Colony-Forming Cells among Spleen Colonies,' which was published in *Journal of Cellular and Comparative Physiology*.

The papers were not instant successes even within the hematology and biophysics communities. 'Spleen colony formation was not widely accepted immediately,' wrote McCulloch, addressing the reaction to the breakthrough papers in his book about the OCI. 'Early attempts to replicate the Toronto method failed.'[20]

Till remembers 'comments on the grapevine that people were having trouble replicating the assay' and that he dealt personally with Stanford University's Robert Kallman. 'He was part of [a] group working with Henry Kaplan, the big-time radiation oncologist who played a major role in changing the treatment for Hodgkin's disease. [Note: A Canadian, Toronto's Dr Vera Peters, was the other person who played a major role.[21]] They were having trouble and I asked him when their mice were dying. He said before ten days. Well, you don't see much before ten days – before the colonies are big enough that you can see them clearly.'

Till's solution was simple: use healthier mice. He wasn't rattled that others couldn't immediately reproduce the results. There was no second-guessing. 'We knew we had it right. We ran the experiments over and over again.'

The next effort – the first for which they actually used the term 'stem cell' in the title – was a Till-driven exercise in using a stochastic approach to statistics to explain variations in the peculiar distribution of colony-forming units in individual spleen colonies, observed in the experiments described in the 1963 paper led by Siminovitch. Basically, stochastics allows for a certain degree of randomness to be factored into statistical calculations. Given that Till and McCulloch were dealing with living cells that were choosing whether to replicate themselves or become blood-forming precursors, a certain amount of randomness was to be expected. Early attempts at computer simulations backed up the stochastic-based analysis.

The response, however, wasn't entirely positive. McCulloch, showing his flair for all things droll, described the mixed reaction: 'Controversy is seldom avoided, particularly when a field moves quickly in response to a new method. Spleen colony formation was no exception.'[22]

The main critic was John J. Trentin from the Division of Experimental Biology at Baylor College of Medicine in Houston. In a paper published in *American Journal of Pathology,* he rejected the stochastic theory by declaring that 'data will be presented indicating that the decision is not random but rather is highly directed' and then constructing his own model of 'hemopoietic inductive microenvironments' or 'HIM.' In essence, Trentin felt that the environment in which the stem cells exist determines how they differentiate.[23]

'We had public conversations at several meetings,' says Till. 'I found it kind of amusing. Biologists have a problem with randomness. They think deterministically. They don't like probability. Whereas someone with [a] physics background, especially if they've studied quantum theory or even nuclear decay, is accustomed to randomness that's mind-boggling.

'I didn't take it personally. It was professional disagreement. I figured it would sort itself out. You can't get too married to models. They're just models. They're designed to explain experimental results. My model was trying to clarify the peculiar distribution of colony-forming units in individual spleen colonies. It was a very strange distribution, with a few colonies producing an awful lot of colony-forming units, then a tailing off to produce very few. The theories aren't mutually exclusive.'

Other researchers built on the work Till and McCulloch had done and took it further – just as they themselves were building on the cutting-edge science of the time. A group of biophysicists in Harwell in England repeated the Becker-led experiments and came up with a novel finding. 'It didn't refute our work, it supplemented it,' says Till. 'They found that if you looked at a lot of spleen colonies, you would find some that had the identical markers in them. If the marked cells had proliferated to some extent before they landed in the spleen you could get more than one colony from the same founder cell. That was interesting, but it didn't negate any of our findings. They published their results in a letter to *Nature* in 1968.'[24]

In fact, if it hadn't been for interaction with the UK group, the 1963 *Nature* paper would never have been possible. 'Charles Ford from Harwell visited us at the OCI and gave a seminar. That was very valuable to us. That was prior to Andy Becker's work. The realization that you could generate chromosomal markers that would persist in viable cells was the basis for the design of Andy's experiment. If we hadn't known about their work we wouldn't have been able to do it.'

True to the OCI credo of looking beyond Canadian borders, McCulloch was eager to exchange knowledge with the best thinkers in the rest of the world. He made a point of attending the annual conferences at Atlantic City, New Jersey, that had been organized for the world's top experimental hematologists by a leading American radiobiologist, Charles Congdon of the Oak Ridge National Laboratory in Tennessee. McCulloch said that after the spleen colony discoveries, he 'was often called upon to report OCI research,' and that the exchanges 'began to change the marrow transplantation/radiation protection field toward clonal analysis and quantitative biology.'[25]

The findings have stood the test of time. As Evelyn Strauss noted in 2005 regarding the pioneering work that earned them the Lasker Award – the most prestigious prize in medical research short of the Nobel – Till and McCulloch, after years of 'ingenious and elegant experiments,' had demonstrated the existence of stem cells:

> They established the properties of stem cells, which still hold true today. Furthermore, they lay the foundation for the isolation of stem cells and for the detection of proteins that help these precursor cells develop and mature. Till and McCulloch's discoveries explained the basis of bone marrow transplantation, which prolongs the lives of patients with leukemia and other cancers of the blood. Moreover, the team set a new standard of rigour for the field of hematology, transforming it from an observational science to a quantitative experimental discipline.[26]

Their 1961 and 1963 papers have been cited thousands of times by researchers who have followed in their footsteps. And they continued to strengthen their case in subsequent papers.

And they continue to inspire others to this day. In late 2010, just months short of the fiftieth anniversary of the 1961 paper, Mick Bhatia, Director of McMaster University's Stem Cell and Cancer Research Institute, published a paper in *Nature* that proved that blood – enough of it for transfusions – can be derived from a patient's own adult skin stem cells. Almost exactly five decades after Till and McCulloch used blood to prove the existence of stem cells, Bhatia reversed their approach and used adult skin stem cells to create blood.

'I still have those papers on my desk,' says Bhatia. 'The 1963 one in *Nature* and the 1961 paper that was the prelude to it. I look at [the *Nature* paper] all the time. It's a classic. Their approach to the science, not knowing anything going in, and how they went at it in a completely non-biased fashion, it's just very artistic. I actually use it as a tool when I have postdocs and students who are venturing into new areas and asking new questions. That work transcends stem cells. It's about how to do everything right when you're exploring unknown biological systems.'

Ripples and Waves

In the field of health research, the work that Till and McCulloch did in the 1960s and into the 1970s has had two major impacts. The first was on hematology, where the effects were immense and almost immediate (after the initial tepid response to the 1961 paper). The second impact, on regenerative medicine, has been no less important and may prove to be even more significant – it has just been slower developing.

Irving Weissman, Director of the Stanford Institute of Stem Cell Biology and Regenerative Medicine, says that it's crucial to remember that many of the concepts now taken for granted about how the body makes blood were still a complete mystery when Till and McCulloch set to work on lumps of cells from irradiated mouse spleens. 'The real discovery,' he says, 'was to turn thinking around from, "The bone marrow is a black box; we don't know anything about it," to, "The bone marrow has discrete cells that can make multiple different cell types."'

Weissman was a medical student when he read the 1961 Till and McCulloch paper 'in a little tiny journal, *Radiation Research*, that had nothing to do with most people.' He remembers it as a defining moment. 'That was a bolt of lightning for me. It said right away that there were these cells in the bone marrow that at the single-cell level could give rise to spleen colonies that had several different blood cell types in them. Nobody had shown or even thought of a single cell having multiple blood cell potentials before that.'

For Weissman, the discovery came out of left field. 'It wasn't in anybody's thinking to look for it. Bone marrow makes blood – that's what we knew. We knew from 1956 on that in a bone marrow transplant, it's the donor cell that gives rise to blood in the recipient. But nobody had asked whether there was one cell in the bone marrow that was a stem cell for T cells [a type of white blood cell crucial to the immune system] or another one that was a stem cell for B cells [another type of white blood cell that's key to fighting off infection] or another one that was a stem cell for red cells [which deliver oxygen to tissue]. Or if there might be common stem or progenitor cell. Now, of course, the spleen colonies don't measure T-lymphocytes or B-lymphocytes; but what they could show is megakaryocytes [large bone marrow cells with nuclei that give rise to blood platelets for coagulation], red blood cells and infection-fighting granulocytes [white blood cells with granules outside the nuclei] and macrophages [scavenger cells that engulf dead, dying, and aberrant cells and infectious agents in all tissues] all came from the same cell.'

What Till and McCulloch accomplished, Weissman says, was to reset how people thought about blood, that vital source of life. 'The whole thing and the whole idea and the set of thinking was you don't think of bone marrow forming each of the blood cells individually from beginning to end, but you think of a hierarchy from stem cells to multi-potent progenitors, to various multiple-lineage progenitors.'

If Till and McCulloch proved the existence of stem cells, Weissman pinpointed their presence: in 1988 he isolated the blood-forming stem cell in mice and followed that up by isolating the human hematopoietic stem cell.

In some ways, Weissman had it easier: he benefited from the pioneering work that his Stanford colleague Leonard Herzenberg had done in developing cell-sorting technology that spared researchers from the tiring and time-consuming task of counting cells under a microscope. 'We could use the cell sorter to combine with the knowledge of what Till and McCulloch had done to begin the search for the stem cell, and that allowed my lab to be the first to do what's called a prospective isolation of the stem cell. But it would have been very difficult for anybody to even start to approach how you would isolate a stem cell if there was no evidence the stem cell existed.'

Weissman was one of many around the world who watched what

Till and McCulloch were doing and who then applied their findings to advance their own work. Australia's Donald Metcalf led the way in developing specialized culture techniques to grow blood cells. That, in turn, led to his discovery of colony-stimulating factors – hormones that determine how white blood cell are formed. This work, for which Metcalf won the Lasker Award in 1993, has helped speed cancer patients' recovery after chemotherapy or radiation treatments.

'The colony-forming units work had a major impact on the thinking of all cellular hematologists, with its demonstration of the clonality and relatedness of disparate hematopoietic populations,' Metcalf wrote in an e-mail from his lab at the Walter and Eliza Hall Institute of Medical Research in Melbourne. 'When we found that our colonies were clonal, we certainly wondered whether they were not formed by the same cells that formed spleen colonies. Events were to show that most *in vitro* colonies were formed by somewhat more mature committed progenitor cells. So the colony-forming units work was certainly close to our minds for many years and indeed remains so.'

Bone Marrow Transplantation

In their enthusiasm for celebrating the discoveries made by Till and McCulloch, some observers have extrapolated that their work directly influenced the Nobel Prize–winning efforts of E. Donnall Thomas in developing bone marrow transplantation techniques. That, says Rainer Storb, a member of the Thomas team since the mid-1960s, would be overstating things.

Thomas reported his first attempt at human bone marrow transplantation in 1957, well before Till and McCulloch made their initial historic find. According to Storb, the early work that Thomas did was linked to several papers published in 1955 and 1956 that 'showed that when you rescued lethally irradiated mice with a spleen cell or a marrow transplant, the rescue was accomplished by cellular elements, by a cell or cells that contributed to the repopulation of marrow spaces.' Storb points to work published by researchers such as Joan M. Main and Richmond T. Prehn of the U.S. National Cancer Institute, John Freeman Loutit and D.W.H. Barnes with the Harwell group in England, and Holland's Dirk van Bekkum as helping build the evidence base for bone marrow transplantation.

'That's what triggered the clinical effort,' says Storb.

Unfortunately, early efforts at bone marrow transplantation – attempted by groups around the world – had been a dismal failure. What had initially worked so well in inbred mice did not translate easily to human beings as clinicians struggled with what came to be known as graft versus host disease. The Thomas team, after its initial foray in 1957, did not attempt another human bone marrow transplantation until the late 1960s, after more than a decade of preclinical research using, primarily, dogs as test subjects. Dogs, says Storb, 'because it's the only species that has the same kind of phenotypic diversity and well-mixed gene pool than humans have.'

'It took a while,' he adds, 'and then we began clinical transplantation in 1968 or 1969 and of course, ran into numerous problems. But we still have patients alive from 1970 or 1971.'

The work that Thomas initiated is being carried forward by his team at the Fred Hutchinson Cancer Research Center in Seattle. 'To this day we're trying to improve on outcomes,' says Storb. 'It's a continuous process.'

Ultimately, the impact of the Till and McCulloch discoveries on the Thomas team's work was more theoretical than technical, says Storb. 'It was the intellectual underpinning for our work. The concept of transplantable marrow cells that were self-replicating was already there at that time. Till and McCulloch's contribution was to document that this originated truly in a single cell. It was a very helpful piece of work. It showed that it's a hierarchical system. It really triggered a lot of the subsequent stem cell work.'

It shouldn't go unobserved, however, that McCulloch was one of the world's earliest innovators in bone marrow transplantation. In the early days at the OCI, he provided the research support for the institute's first transplant attempts involving terminally ill children. Writing about himself in the third person in his book about the OCI, McCulloch explains:

> A novel clinical feature of the hospital was a special ward for the treatment of children with cancer. The first pediatrician was John Darte. Fully trained in pediatrics, Darte spent two years in Manchester, learning radiation therapy ... He readily formed collaborative links. With the help of McCulloch he performed three marrow transplants as a treatment for leukemia in children. These were certainly the first human transplants in Canada and may have been the first in the world. One temporary remis-

sion was obtained. Unfortunately, the early experience was discouraging and was reported only orally at a meeting. Darte left the OCI to go to Newfoundland, and soon the pediatric ward was closed.[27]

McCulloch is off the mark in suggesting that these were 'certainly the first human transplants in Canada and may have been the first in the world,' for Thomas had already reported on his efforts in 1957, the same year a transplant was attempted in Regina in an unsuccessful effort to save a fifty-one-year-old farmer who was dying of chronic lymphatic leukemia.[28] McCulloch also may have the number of transplant attempts incorrect: Hans Messner, Director of the Bone Marrow Transplantation Program at the Princess Margaret Hospital, suggests that starting in 1960 there were five transplants done at the Princess Margaret Hospital by McCulloch and Darte. Regardless, the evidence is clear that McCulloch was responsible for the early attempts in the then highly experimental therapy. He would go on to lead the program when the OCI re-established bone marrow transplantation in 1970.

Storb, who is from Germany, became involved in bone marrow transplantation partly due to McCulloch. 'I met him for the first time when I was still working in Paris in 1963 or 1964. There was a meeting at which I heard him make a presentation. I found McCulloch vibrant and intellectual and charismatic. It was additional impetus to draw me into the field. That's when I first got interested in this and joined Don Thomas's lab.'

Embryonic Stem Cells

Besides significantly advancing the understanding of hematology, and providing the underpinning for bone marrow transplantation as a therapy for leukemia and other blood-based disorders, the work that Till and McCulloch did has proven to be of fundamental importance to the development of regenerative medicine.

'Every so often you get these conceptual leaps about how biological processes work,' says Sir John Bell, the ex-pat Canadian who is now Regius Chair of Medicine at Oxford University and the President of the Academy of Medical Sciences. 'Although the concepts of tissue repair and regeneration and development had existed as individual entities before 1961, the concept that you had discrete cell populations that populated and self-renewed, which was ultimately their breakthrough, changed the way everybody thought about that particular discipline. If you take the broad field of regenerative medicine ... Till and McCulloch are obviously pretty central to the evolution of that field. Although it took a further twenty or thirty years for the field to really take off, those were very much the seminal observations that set it on its course.'

In fact, it took something completely beyond Till and McCulloch's blood-based discoveries to trigger the explosion of interest in stem cell research and regenerative medicine. That 'something' was the isolation of human embryonic stem cells by James Thomson at the University of Wisconsin in 1998.

'The discovery of human embryonic stem cells has captivated the world,' says Alan Bernstein, past President of the Canadian Institutes of Health Research, who now leads the Global HIV Vaccine Enterprise. 'But that's a completely different field than hematopoietic stem cells. The basic context and definition and criteria for what you call stem cells were established by Till and McCulloch. Whether everybody working on embryonic stem cells knows this, I'm not sure.'

Research into embryonic stem cells was going on in parallel with the work Till and McCulloch and others were doing in hematology. Its roots trace back to the 1950s, to investigations undertaken by Leroy Stevens at the Jackson Laboratory in Bar Harbor, Maine. Stevens was investigating the properties of teratomas – 'monster' tumours that occur primarily in the male testis or female ovaries and that can grow to include both undifferentiated cells and differentiated ones for things like hair and bone.

'What he discovered was that these tumours came from germ cells, from primordial germ cells that began to proliferate in an abnormal way in the embryonic testis and then developed into these tumours with a striking variety of differentiated cell types,' says Gail Martin, a leader in developmental biology at the University of California, San Francisco. 'So he had the idea that the primordial germ cells were pluripotent, which wasn't a leap, and that they could start to grow and proliferate abnormally and then differentiate.'

Stevens developed a strain of mice with a very high predisposition for the cancerous tumours more commonly known as teratocarcinomas. That enabled the work to be carried forward by him and others, including Americans Lewis Kleinsmith and Barry Pierce, who in 1964 published proof that a single teratocarcinoma cell, also known as an embryonal carcinoma cell, could give rise to all the cells in these tumours.[29] It snowballed from there. Throughout the 1970s, researchers studied teratocarcinomas to unlock the mystery of how to isolate stem cells directly from the tumours and subsequently from mouse embryos. Martin, who coined the term 'embryonic stem cell,' was one of the first to accomplish the feat, in 1981.

'It took five years, basically,' says Martin. 'Unbeknownst to me, Martin Evans [her former postdoctoral supervisor] was doing the same thing at Cambridge University. We both discovered how to isolate stem cells directly from embryos. I came up with the term "embryonic stem cells" to distinguish them from embryonal carcinoma cells.'

Evans went on to be knighted and to share the Nobel Prize in Physiology or Medicine in 2007 with Mario R. Capecchi and Oliver Smithies (a geneticist who spent his early years as a researcher, from 1954 to 1960, at the University of Toronto) after introducing specific gene modifications in 'knockout mice' using embryonic stem cells. Martin, widely regarded as one of the top regenerative medicine researchers in the world, says that while she read the Till and McCulloch papers, they were background information to her work in embryonic stem cells. 'The work was there, but it wasn't really the focus.'

As Bernstein says, it was Thomson's isolation of human embryonic stem cells in 1998 that sparked worldwide interest in stem cells and caught the public's imagination. As reported on the front page of the *Washington Post*:

> The long-awaited discovery of the so-called, human embryonic stem cells – the primordial human cells that give rise to all the specialized tissues in a developing fetus – was hailed by researchers as a landmark event with vast biomedical potential. The cells multiply tirelessly in laboratory dishes, offering a self-replenishing supply from which scientists hope to grow replacement tissues for people with various diseases, including bone marrow for cancer patients, neurons for people with Alzheimer's diseases and pancreatic cells for people with diabetes.[30]

But while embryonic stem cell research was being carried out separately from what Till and McCulloch had done at the OCI, it caused many to take a fresh look at what they had accomplished and apply it to their work.

Samuel Weiss, the Canadian researcher who discovered neural stem cells, says that it all loops back to Till and McCulloch. His own investigations have borrowed heavily from assays they designed with blood-based stem cells thirty years earlier.

'It just was so profound. In terms of its impact and understanding of the potential of self-renewal, proliferation, differentiation, all of this sort of biology emerged from their pioneering work. I still remind people that if it hadn't been [for] hematopoietic stem cells and their biology, all other stem cell biology would probably have yet to be discovered.'

PART TWO

Development

4

A Bunch of Kids Having a Good Time

Jim Till remembers an annual general meeting of the Stem Cell Network, held a few years ago in Montreal, at which he and Ernest McCulloch were honoured. Both gave speeches to the stem cell scientists – young and old – from across Canada who had assembled in the hall.

'Alan Bernstein was chairing the session,' says Till, 'and after we had spoken, he said, "I want to do a little experiment. I would like to have the people who worked directly with either Till or McCulloch stand up." So a few people stood up, and Alan of course was one of them and he was already standing. And then he said, "I would like the people who have worked with the people who just stood up to stand up." And he kept that up and eventually it was about two-thirds of the room, as I recall.'

The discovery of stem cells by Till and McCulloch has had a lasting impact on health research, but their influence went well beyond pure science. What they did – and the doggedly determined way in which they did it – inspired the generations that came after them. There are hundreds, perhaps thousands, of health researchers and administrators at work across Canada and around the world who, in ways large and small, direct and indirect, have benefited from the work of Till and McCulloch and the example they set. Several, through the discoveries Till and McCulloch nurtured and the leadership qualities they helped hone, went on to become world leaders in medical research in the late twentieth and early twenty-first centuries.

'We were just a bunch of kids having a good time,' says the Ottawa Health Research Institute's Mike McBurney, who did his PhD studies at the OCI in the late 1960s and early 1970s. 'I didn't really appreciate who was there. It was a veritable Who's Who of science today. When I went to Oxford for my postdoc, there were seven Nobel Laureates on the street where I worked. I was a little bit surprised that the people in Toronto were just as clever as the people at Oxford.'

Bernstein was one of those just-as-clever people at the OCI. For most of the first decade of this century, he was the most powerful figure in health research in Canada. The inaugural President of the Canadian Institutes of Health Research (CIHR), Bernstein ran what has become a $1 billion a year agency that supports thousands of researchers across the country. Since leaving the top post at CIHR, he has led the New York–based Global HIV Vaccine Enterprise, which places him in professional circles that include Bill Gates and Bill Clinton. In late 2010, he was nominated by then Governor Arnold Schwarzenegger to be the next chair of the California Institute for Regenerative Medicine, an agency that received $3 billion in funding for stem cell research after it was approved by California voters in 2004. A technicality – Bernstein's lack of American citizenship – prevented him from taking the job that would have made him one of the most influential voices in regenerative medicine in the world.[31]

'For a lot of different reasons it seemed like a great fit,' says Bernstein. 'I wasn't looking for a position and I'm very happy in my current job, but this seemed too good to pass up. Then they found a technicality that you have to be an American citizen. It was very unfortunate because I felt I needed to inform my staff and my board that I was going to allow my name to stand, because it's a very public process. Then three or four days later the whole thing fell apart. It was an unfortunate experience in my career, but it's behind me now. Onwards and upwards.'

Bernstein's upwards climb began on Sherbourne Street, where he toiled first as a undergrad summer student at the OCI, then as a PhD student with Till from 1968 to 1972. After two years of postdoc work in Britain, he returned to the OCI as a staff member. He stayed there for eleven years before leaving to help Lou Siminovitch set up the Samuel Lunenfeld Research Institute at Mount Sinai Hospital. According to Siminovitch, Bernstein helped fashion it into 'an internationally competitive institute in a relatively short time.' The two men eventually fell out when Bernstein replaced Siminovitch as director in 1990. 'Not a happy ending,' Siminovitch writes in his book.[32] Bernstein puts it this way: 'The issues between Lou and I are unfortunate because I always had the highest respect for Lou as human being and a scientist. He was one of my mentors for a good number of years. The problems in our relationship stemmed from me succeeding him. My relationship has not ended. I don't have any meaningful discussions with Lou any more, but certainly when I see him in Toronto we chat politely.'

Bernstein learned from Till how to manage people: 'Jim appreciated that people are all different and they need to be treated as individuals, not as students in a category. He treated me differently than he treated the other three students. I'm not saying better or worse, but as an individual. That's one thing I learned. Another is that running a division the way Jim ran it [Till was head of the OCI's Biological Research Division from 1969 to 1982] is very different than science. It's about people. You have to recruit the very best people and give them a really long leash and let them make their own mistakes, let them make their own successes ... creating the right intellectual environment for them to thrive. Jim was a very hands-off mentor; his ego was not out of line. His job was to make sure you succeeded.'

That Bernstein flourished under Till is not surprising. Like Till, Bernstein came out of a non-biology background, having earned his undergrad degree in mathematics and physics. He is almost proud of the fact that before his time at the OCI, he hadn't taken a biology course since Oakwood Collegiate, where he remembers taking 'a stunningly boring' grade ten class for which he copied his older sister's notes on an assignment about the parts of the flower. 'She got an A. I traced what she had done and I got a B. I think it was because she was a pretty girl and I was a bored guy.'

After completing his Bachelor of Science degree at the University of Toronto, Bernstein knew he didn't want to stay in physics. 'I could see role models like Jim. My background was not that different. There was a resemblance there that really helped me.' Till encouraged Bernstein to pursue his burgeoning interest in genetics even though he himself was not particularly adept in the field and would not be able to supervise the work closely. The hands-off approach worked well: Bernstein did world-class work on tumour viruses, expanding the understanding of the role of the Friend virus in a form of leukemia called erythroleukemia. He has co-authored more than two hundred peer-reviewed articles, ten of which have been published in the prestigious pages of *Nature,* the research equivalent to batting in the World Series or playing in the Stanley Cup Finals. Building on Till and McCulloch's foundations, Bernstein's work has advanced science's understanding of cancer, embryonic development, the cardiovascular system, and the formation of blood cells.

Bernstein now runs a global research operation out of an office on Park Avenue. Yet to this day, he seeks Till's advice. 'When I go to see Jim, I am a graduate student again. There's something comforting about telling him what's on your mind, that you need some advice. He's just a great mentor.'

McCulloch, on the other hand, was always more of an enigma to Bernstein, who recalls how the older man could throw him into a dither with an off-the-cuff comment.

'He had this unique style of being very quick, being a little bit cryptic in his remarks,' Bernstein explains. 'When I was a summer student at the OCI I was trying to purify hematopoietic stem cells. They are roughly one in 10,000 or one in 20,000 cells in our bone marrow, so how do you purify them? One of my projects was to purify away other cell types like macrophages to enrich for stem cells. I was using magnetic particles that macrophages would eat up, then I'd throw a magnet in and the macrophages would stick to the magnets.

'That was the idea anyway – it never really worked. But I had to give a little update to [McCulloch's] spleen team at our weekly meetings, which I did. Bun asked me if I'd read something by Shaw. I was so nervous – he'd put his hand up and made this comment. I had to make a quick decision whether to lie or not. And I said, "No I haven't," and he said, "Well, you should." Later, I asked him, "What's the reference?" And he said, "It's George Bernard Shaw, *The Doctor's Dilemma*."

'I went out and I got the book, the play, and I read through it, and there's one line in there. Another name for a macrophage is a phagocyte. They gobble up stuff, usually germs or in this case the magnetic particles. So there's one line in there where the doctor mentions phagocytes. I had to read that whole bloody play just to find this one line, which was the reason that Bun had referred to it after my presentation. I'll never forget that.'

Bernstein thinks that McCulloch's quirky tendency to pull ideas out of the blue was part of a deliberate strategy to challenge the people around him to think beyond the ordinary. 'What Bun did, that style that he had, it kept all of us on our toes. He must have been aware of it, because it made us all see a way of thinking out of the box. That was his style, an out-of-the-box thinker all of the time.'

Bernstein says that scientists who worked closely with McCulloch often developed a fierce loyalty to him – one that was reciprocated. 'If you worked in Bun's lab, there was a two-way loyalty there which was quite remarkable. Bun would just do anything for you if you worked with him or for him.'

The McCulloch Charisma Factor

A beneficiary of that loyalty is Tak Wah Mak. A colleague of Bernstein's at the OCI in the 1970s and into the 1980s, the two men shared authorship of more than twenty high-profile academic papers. But if Bernstein was primarily a Till devotee during his time at the OCI, Mak was definitely a McCulloch disciple. 'You work with McCulloch,' says Mak, 'you would walk in front of a bus for him. And he would for you.'

Mak's relationship with McCulloch began soon after he arrived at the OCI in 1972 to do postdoctoral work with Rose Sheinin. 'However, that didn't last very long and I got interested in what Dr McCulloch's lab was doing. There was a very fun group of people who were very interested in science and, before you knew it, I was so intrigued that I switched.'

Two years after Mak arrived, it was Till who offered him a job as a Senior Scientist in the Biological Research Division. But Mak could see McCulloch's invisible hand at work in the decision: 'I'm quite confident it was McCulloch and not Till that got me the job, because Till was a very different person. Till was a very meticulous, organized, deep-thinking, logical person. I was not the Till type, because my thoughts are [all] over everywhere. My kind of mental predisposition is closer to McCulloch's than Till's.'

In 1979, after working closely with Bernstein, Mak returned to the University of Wisconsin, where he had earned his bachelor's and master's degrees, to spend a year with Nobel Prize winner Howard Temin. There, he concentrated on molecular biology. He then returned to Toronto and joined McCulloch's leukemia program. 'Everybody took an aspect of leukemia and I took T cell leukemia. From there I got interested in T cell development and T cell receptors and went in that direction.'

Mak gained international attention in 1984 for his discovery of the human T cell receptor and the gene that produces it. T cells (so named because they are generated in the thymus) protect the body from various infections, killing cells that have invader viruses or triggering antibody responses. Finding the T cell receptor opened new doors to understanding recurring infections, cancers, and autoimmune diseases such as AIDS.

He was not alone in this work: Stanford University's Mark Davis, working independently, identified the T cell receptor in mice. But Mak's *Nature* paper, 'A Human T Cell-Specific cDNA Clone Encodes a Protein Having Extensive Homology to Immunoglobulin Chains,'[33] sparked attention around the world. Interestingly, the discovery came from work that few were originally keen to support.

'When we proposed the idea to clone the T cell receptor to the National Cancer Institute of Canada we were basically laughed off,' says Mak. McCulloch would recall that he and other senior OCI scientists 'did not think the National Cancer Institute of Canada reviewers to be infallible'[34] and that they encouraged Mak to carry on.

'The only person that really believed me was McCulloch,' says Mak. 'Some reviewers will tell you, "You are a moron, you don't know what you're doing. This is all wrong." They may have points – they may be right, and you have to learn from them. But they may be wrong. And when they're wrong, and people like McCulloch say, "You know, I think you're right," that can make all the difference in the world. McCulloch was behind me when the rest of the world thought I was crazy. He saw some quality in me. McCulloch bought into me.'

Mak also appreciated McCulloch's ability to focus on the science and ignore the colour of the scientist's skin or his or her religion. 'At the end of the 1970s [at the OCI], there were these two individuals: there was Tak Mak, and there was Alan Bernstein – a Chinese man from Hong Kong and a Jewish boy from Toronto. And the world of science and the world of politics in Toronto were not really, in the 1970s, crazy about embracing either one of us.'

Unlike Bernstein, who transitioned into the executive suite to run health research, Mak has stayed in the lab and published prodigiously. Over four decades, his name has appeared on more than 650 papers and letters, including 30-plus *Nature* articles. It's not just about volume: in 2000, *ScienceWatch* ranked him one of the top ten scientists in the world based on the number of highly cited reports he had produced in the previous two years.[35] He also has more than thirty-five patents granted or pending. But unlike his mentor, Mak – who studied as a chemical engineer before switching to biochemistry – has moved about in medical research and refers to himself as a 'scientific vagabond.'

After developing 'knockout mice' with a specific gene or specific genes missing, in 1989 Mak set out to advance the new technology to better understand genes' roles and functions in diseases. His work drew the interest of Amgen, the California-based biotechnology giant, which in 1993 agreed to create a research institute, the OCI-affiliated Amgen Institute, with Mak as its director. He held that post until 2002, when he shifted his interest to breast cancer – the disease that had claimed his wife in 1998 – and created the Advanced Medical Discovery Institute.

'I had guilt for two years. I couldn't even look myself in the mirror for two years, thinking that I could have spent more time with her, that we were waiting for the days we would retire.' He is also Director of the Campbell Family Institute for Breast Cancer Research at the Princess Margaret Hospital.

Not slowing down, in 2009 Mak secured a multimillion-dollar, four-year grant through the Cancer Stem Cell Consortium to co-lead a Californian/Canadian project to identify and develop new drugs to target cells that initiate solid tumour cancers. 'I'll be sixty-five [in 2011] and I should be retired, but there is absolutely no question in my mind I will have another five or ten years,' says Mak, who throughout his career has turned down frequent offers from some of the leading research centres in the world.

'After the T cell, I was really, really hot. It was Harvard, it was Yale. People in Stanford said, "You know, we can cook something up for you, too." And the Max Planck Institute in Germany. Basically, I could have had a lot of jobs.'

Beyond the roots he had put down in the biomedical community in Toronto, Mak points to McCulloch as an important reason for staying in Canada. 'Absolutely. My loyalty to him.' He particularly remembers coming back to the OCI after deciding not to take a prestigious position at Yale:

'The next day I told McCulloch that I wanted to come back, could he sweeten the deal for me, so that I can stay? And McCulloch said, "Are you trying to tell me I should buy that piece of equipment that you requested last year, that I'd given up because I thought you were gone?" And then he said, "What else do you want?" I looked at him and I said to myself, "Tak, just settle for anything. Everybody saves face, you want to be here, you don't want to go, don't try for anything more." And you know what I did? I wanted a key to the back door of the hospital. The parking lot was at the back. On weekends and evenings, you'd park at the back and you had to walk all around the hospital to get to the front. You had a key to the back door, you could come through. That's what I got.'

His loyalty to McCulloch was based on more than shared experiences in the science lab. He regarded McCulloch, two decades his senior, as both a friend and a father figure. His own father had abandoned his family when Mak was only four.

'We are very, very close,' he said in an interview before McCulloch's death. 'We are as different as we can be. I am a Chinese from Hong

Kong. I grew up in the United States and still speak English with an accent. I still think in terms of Confucianism, Taoism. And then there's McCulloch, a Canadian gentleman and scholar of Scottish descent, as eccentric as you can be, and quotes Shakespeare, Jane Austen, Keats, and Wordsworth. We couldn't be any more different. But he adopted my family into his family. We lived one block away from each other. His wife Ona loved our family. When my wife died, his wife gave the eulogy.'

Mak also recognizes that McCulloch could be a frustrating authority figure. 'Some secretaries would go crazy under him. They would come and talk to me and go, "What's wrong with the guy? He doesn't even say thank you! I killed myself all weekend to finish this grant for him." And I would say, "You don't need to hear him say thank you, you just know that he is grateful."'

If many found McCulloch to be an intimidating force, Mak, who is cut from the same random-synapse intellectual cloth as his mentor, was not. 'Science is about connections. There are thousands of these rocks, and you remember that on October 5, 1998, you turned over a rock on the other side of the mountain and it fits the piece of rock that you're holding in your hand now. It comes from a lot of experience, it comes from a lot of connections in your brain, it comes from having seen and read a lot. McCulloch, he was able to make those connections. I never felt intimidated. I just hit it off at the personal level. He is a very charismatic and brilliant original thinker.'

The New Beginning of Bone Marrow Transplantation

If McCulloch's charisma could help keep research talent like Tak Mak from leaving Canada, it could also convince a hot young prospect to come to the country. Hans Messner, who would go on to become Director of the Bone Marrow Transplantation Program at the Princess Margaret Hospital, was a medical student in Freiburg, Germany, when he was assigned the task of picking McCulloch up at the airport in Basel, Switzerland, and delivering him to a stem cell conference.

'On the way to the conference in Freiburg we had quite a nice discussion. I spent quite a bit of time with him during the meeting and he asked about my thesis work. At the end of the meeting, he comes by and says "It's all set – I talked to your supervisor and you're going to come to Toronto." I said, "I am? Okay, fine." That's why I'm here. I didn't have any say. I was twenty-seven. I wasn't married. I came here in 1969. I met my wife the first day I set foot in the Princess Margaret Hospital. It was definitely destiny.'

In truth, long before the airport meeting Messner was well aware of the work that Till and McCulloch had done. He knew all about the colony-forming units, and as a doctor in training who routinely saw leukemia patients dying in the cancer ward, he was keen to learn more about bone marrow transplantation. 'McCulloch told me all about the work that they were doing. It was all new territory. To me it was like going to a toy store. I really wanted to do that.'

In the late 1960s, McCulloch, having collaborated with pediatrician John Darte on some of the world's earliest attempts at human bone marrow transplantation, was eager to get a program going again.

'If you really go back in the history, there was a total of six [Canadian] transplants done well before that,' says Messner. 'The first one was in 1957 in Regina, Saskatchewan. Then, starting in 1960 and 1961, there were five transplants done at the Princess Margaret Hospital and Dr McCulloch and Dr Darte did those transplants. That was what we would call the pre-scientific era of transplantation. They had no human leukocyte antigen typing, which is basically the prerequisite to determine compatibility between two individuals. These were very early. Globally, some two hundred transplants were done and then things fizzled by about 1962 because the prerequisites weren't established.'

According to Messner, Canada's first 'new sequence' bone marrow transplantation took place at the Princess Margaret Hospital on 10 June 1970. 'I was part of that. There was a group of individuals. Of course, Dr McCulloch. Dr Don Cowan was the clinical lead. Then there were two members who did an interesting experimental component of it – Bob Phillips and Rick Miller. They had developed a technology trying, for the first time, to separate cells that could cause graft versus host disease from the stem cell population that would be repopulating the marrow.'

Messner's records show that the history-making team included Daniel Bergsagel and Bill Rider, the Chiefs of Medical and Radiation Oncology at Princess Margaret, along with Richard Hasselback, John Senn, Victor Fornasier, Hakam Abu-Zahra, Dominick Amato, Bertie Aye, Albert Clarysse, Abdul Ragab, and Norman Iscove.

But it was McCulloch, says Messner, who was the force behind the first Canadian bone marrow transplantation program. 'He was the overall lead, particularly scientifically. It started out as being his program and he made sure that all the resources were put together so we could do these kinds of things. He was the big leader – he needs to get that credit. The fourth transplant, which was done in 1972, was our first long-term survivor. This person died in 2004. So, thirty-two years. It's nearly two thousand of those transplants that we have done.'

Those figures are just for the allogenic transplants involving stem cells donated from a genetically similar donor. The technology for autologous bone marrow transplantation – using the patient's own bone marrow – was developed in the 1980s.

'The autologous program in Toronto really started under a different idea,' says Messner. 'In the old Princess Margaret Hospital [on Sherbourne Street, before relocation to University Avenue] we had no space to accommodate that. At that time it was Ken Shumak who was working at the Toronto General Hospital to try and set that up. We helped him with it. He moved on academically and it was then Dr Armand Keating who started to build the autologous program in the mid-1980s. In 1998 there was the merger that formed the University Health Network and all the activity, including the autologous program, moved over to the Princess Margaret Hospital. The number for autologous is higher than the one for allogenic transplants.'

The bone marrow transplantation successes at the Princess Margaret Hospital had been 'directly spawned' by the Till and McCulloch discoveries, says Messner. 'This is a translational arm of the basic science. I was fortunate enough to be around at the time when this was starting to ferment properly and we were able to start to do the first successful transplants.'

Till and McCulloch also had a significant impact on bone marrow transplantation in British Columbia, where the husband-and-wife team of Allen Eaves, a former PhD student with the OCI's Robert Bruce, and Connie Eaves, the former Till postdoc, relocated in the 1970s.

'After Connie and I moved out to Vancouver,' says Allen Eaves, 'there was a national competition to set up bone marrow transplant programs in centres across Canada and I wrote a proposal. I was a newly minted oncology–hematology type trying to stimulate some of my colleagues to set up a bone marrow transplantation program. At the time we were linking the hematopoietic concepts of stem cells that Till and McCulloch developed with bone marrow transplantation – the clinical application of these concepts.'

According to Eaves, the proposal, submitted in 1979 on behalf of the Vancouver General Hospital and the British Columbia Cancer Agency, received provincial funding that initiated the Leukemia/Bone Marrow Transplantation Program of British Columbia.

They scored a breakthrough. The Eaves co-authored a paper in the *New England Journal of Medicine* in 1983 showing that when the bone marrow of a patient with chronic myelogenous leukemia was placed in culture flasks for ten days, the leukemic stem cells died off and normal hematopoietic stem cells started to grow out. 'We called it "culture purging,"' says Allen Eaves, 'and it was quite a revolutionary concept because the thinking then was there were no normal hematopoietic stem cells left in chronic myelogenous leukemia patients; rather, they'd all been squeezed out by the huge number of leukemia cells present in the marrow of these patients at diagnosis.'

Since most patients don't have a tissue-matched, compatible sibling donor for an allogenic bone marrow transplant, this discovery meant that culture purging could be used to prepare a patient's own marrow, free of leukemic cells, for an autologous transplant. Over the next decade, he estimates, about sixty autologous bone marrow transplants on chronic myelogenous leukemia patients were carried out in Vancouver using the process. 'These were patients who were otherwise going to die. And the survival rate was about 50 per cent. So this was exciting stuff.'

These clinical studies showed that normal hematopoietic stem cells could be separated from leukemic stem cells and that normal stem cells could be manipulated for many days outside the body and then put back into patients where they would grow normally – a necessity for the evolving fields of tissue engineering and regenerative medicine. Eaves says that this research work helped attract American transplant specialist Gordon L. Phillips to Vancouver in 1984.

In 1985, Eaves was appointed Head of Clinical Hematology at the Vancouver General Hospital and the University of British Columbia, with the goal of building a world-class clinical hematology program and linking it to the outstanding basic science research ongoing in the Terry Fox Lab, an institution that has been seminal in furthering many of the concepts developed by Till and McCulloch. 'We were really one of the first transplant programs in Canada,' he says, 'one of the first to really get going. In all, by the early 1990s we had treated about 1,200 or 1,300 patients.'

Those transplants, he says, track back to what he learned at the OCI.

'Absolutely,' says Eaves, who was founding Director of the Terry Fox Lab and who also created a thriving bioscience reagents and tools company called STEMCELL Technologies Inc. 'There is no question that what Till and McCulloch laid out were the concepts for understanding stem cells – specifically, how they grow and differentiate and how these cellular processes are perturbed in cancer. It was seminal.'

Till's Eye for Talent

Like McCulloch, Till was no slouch in attracting talent to the OCI. One of his biggest coups was landing Victor Ling, a former OCI summer student in his undergrad years who was beginning his career in molecular biology. By 1971, after completing a postdoc with Cambridge's Fred Sanger (who by then had already won one Nobel Prize and would go on to win a second), Ling had the credentials to establish his own lab anywhere in the world.

'I met Jim at some meeting back in Canada,' says Ling. 'He asked how I was doing, because we knew each other from when I was a summer student. I asked him if there were any positions and he goes, "Yeah." I asked, "Well could I have one?" He just looked at me and said, "You've got it." Jim wasn't questioning. He didn't say I'd have to go for an interview or anything like that. He simply asked me when I wanted to start. I don't think I ever actually had a contract.'

Working at the OCI in 1974, Ling identified p-glycoprotein, a protein that pushes substances out of cells and plays a key role in multi-drug resistance – a significant advance in oncology. The Vancouver-based Ling is now President and Scientific Director of the Terry Fox Research Institute. He recalls that his time at the OCI was particularly satisfying. 'People were really focused on wanting to make discoveries. There was also a feeling that one could do anything there. There was no restriction in the imagination or aspiration to want to do things. There was kind of a feeling that, you know, anything's possible.'

Bob Phillips was another Till recruit. He grew up in the United States and did his PhD in the early 1960s at Washington University in St Louis, where he read about what Till and McCulloch were doing at the OCI in the early *Radiation Research* papers. 'I was just fascinated with the way they had done it, so I started following all their papers and waiting for them to come out.'

Phillips wrote to Till and got hired in 1965 as a postdoctoral fellow, planning to stay in Canada for two years. Instead, he had a twenty-one-year run at the OCI, rising to the position of Chairman of the Department of Medical Biophysics. He and colleague Rick Miller devised an apparatus called STAPUT to sort cells in an effort to improve the odds of avoiding graft versus host disease in bone marrow transplantation

– an innovation that helped launch the bone marrow transplantation program at the Princess Margaret Hospital in 1970. He also did seminal work in furthering science's understanding of retinoblastomas, which are hereditary tumours of the eye that occur mainly in young children. Phillips left the OCI in 1986 to become Director of Research for Hematology/Oncology at Toronto's Hospital for Sick Children. He went on to become President of the National Cancer Institute of Canada in 1994; he was named its Executive Director two years later, a post he held for five years. Phillips postponed retirement in 2010 to take a two-year posting as the CEO of the Integrated BioBank of Luxembourg.

Phillips remembers McCulloch fondly. 'I knew him when he was a faculty member and he had a few strange traits, but I know others that are a lot stranger. He was always chewing on chalk, so he had this smudge on the corner of his mouth. He would get frustrated and throw his chalk at the chalkboard – or at you if you frustrated him.'

That notwithstanding, McCulloch was a friendly – if chalk-smudged – face at the OCI for Phillips. 'Oh absolutely. His door was always open and you could go down and talk to him about anything.' He regards McCulloch as one of the most interesting people he has ever met. 'He was just constantly innovating, seeing new ways of doing things.'

Like Bernstein, Phillips continued to seek advice from Till long after leaving the OCI. 'He's been very helpful in the last ten years. I'd bounce ideas off of him and say, "What do you know about this? What do you think about that?"'

What he learned from Till and McCulloch was to take 'a broader approach to things. To try to keep my mind open to other interpretations, not to be afraid of new technology – because they were always early adopters of new technology. They were very quick to establish collaborations both inside and outside of Toronto, always looking to see what other people were doing and what we could learn from them. They also taught me how to write papers. They taught me how to run a laboratory. What I learned and practised later on, I picked up at the OCI.'

Simon Sutcliffe came to the OCI from the United Kingdom in 1979 to get two years of training in radiation oncology. He ended up staying seventeen years and became its President and CEO in 1994. A good way to understand Till, he says, is to look at the career of Alastair Cunningham, who was working in immunology while Till was heading the OCI's Division of Biological Research.

'Alastair was a hardcore immunologist,' says Sutcliffe. 'He'd written textbooks, he established publications, [he was] a senior figure in immunobiology. And for whatever reason, Alastair decided that he would actually go into complementary and alternative medicine. That's quite a shift, if you can imagine ... a move from hardcore immunobiology and the studies of the T cell and all the various other things that go along with it, to, "I'm now going to devote myself to complementary medicine and how patients can be supported and how beliefs in health will influence outcome, and take a sort of more esoteric, hypothetical, neurobiological frame to how I will stare at my future."

'Alastair's been in that business now since 1985 or so and has probably become one of the leading figures in behavioural science as it relates to cancer patients. Now, Jim was totally supportive of that move. You know, there might be many who would say, "I hired you as a hardcore immunologist, I'm not interested in you being a flaky complementary scientist." But I think Jim's thinking – and I'm hypothesizing here – is if you're going to do something well enough and apply science to it and rigour, it doesn't matter what you do, something will come out as credible answers.'

Cunningham agrees. 'Jim was very supportive. He's that kind of man. I remember thinking that this was what I had to do, because of various things in my own life. I realized that my immunology wasn't helping anybody very much and [that] I had to shift to something that was going to be of direct relevance to cancer patients. And this was a growing interest of mine. Jim was immediately willing to support me. He never raised any objection and he allowed me to do a second PhD as a sort of sabbatical and retain my job as I was doing it. So I'm very grateful to him.'

McCulloch, on the other hand, was anything but supportive. When he succeeded Till as division head, he saw Cunningham's move to cancer psychology as 'a problem.' He felt that 'Cunningham's protocol did not have enough research rigour' and went so far as to restrict his annual salary increase 'as much as possible.'[36]

Despite this, Cunningham carried on his investigations into the role of the mind and its effect on quality of life and survival in cancer patients. He flourished. Appointed an Officer of the Order of Canada in 2003, he was a co-winner of the first Dr Rogers Prize for Excellence in Complementary and Alternative Medicine in 2007, sharing the $250,000 prize with Victoria's Dr Abram Hoffer.

Cunningham declined to be quoted about McCulloch, beyond saying that 'he was never very understanding of what I was doing. Apart from cutting back a bit of salary, he didn't do me much harm.' Of Till, he can't say enough good: 'He's a real straight arrow. Just a wonderful, straight-talking guy. Not a devious bone in his body. He was an excellent head of the department and encouraging to everyone, not just me.'

Says Sutcliffe: 'Within the OCI, [Till] had recruited some really stellar people into positions in which they really embellished their reputations. Recognizing that they obviously have inherent intelligence and talent, I have absolutely no doubt they were all shaped by Jim's open declaration of the rigour of science. The characteristic of that rigour is: whatever you do, you actually have to do it with a level of credibility and respect that immediately puts you at the advancing edge of the field.'

Till, not big on self-aggrandizement, nonetheless knows his strengths. 'I flatter myself in this one way: I think I'm not a bad judge of talent.'

One of the reasons Till understood Cunningham's desire to change fields was his own decision to move on. In 1980, he began walking away from stem cell research. McCulloch had shifted his interest to leading the bone marrow transplantation program for leukemia patients. As a physicist, Till didn't feel comfortable or qualified in this area. 'To contribute to human work you really need to be able to work with patients, you need an MD, and I didn't have one. I felt I didn't have much to contribute. We had regular rounds where we talked with the basic scientists and the clinicians. I remember being taken aback at being asked advice about how to deal with a particular patient. I thought, "I shouldn't be commenting on this." I simply didn't see what I would be contributing as a non-physician. All I could do was statistical stuff and I didn't want to become a statistical analyst.'

Another reason for leaving the field he had founded was recognition that he needed to step aside to let the next generations take over. 'The model had been to try to get students and postdocs who were better than you were. We succeeded. A number of people who had come through the group were out on their own in 1980. I had great respect for them, they were really good. I didn't want to compete with them for funding. I wanted them to move ahead. I thought, "I've done what I can do in his area."'

He had also become interested in a completely different area of health research: quantifying the quality of life of cancer patients. 'I knew from my experience with radiotherapy, with radiotherapists and with clinicians in the treatment of leukemia, that quite often what was actually delivered was not a cure but improvement of quality of life. So, shouldn't that be measured? Can you measure quality of life? Shouldn't that be part of one of the endpoints used in clinical trials?

'I discovered that the psychologists had been doing a lot of work on questionnaires to assess aspects of quality of life, like pain, with quite sophisticated methods. At that point I hooked up with Norman Boyd, a breast cancer specialist who had joined the OCI. We decided to start a group studying quality of life and how that could be incorporated into medical decision making. And away we went. We were some of the earliest people working in it. For patients, quality of life matters a great deal.'

Till has had to cope with bouts of depression in his life, something he is reluctant to talk about because of the stigma that persists around mental illness. While he says this heightened his sensitivity to quality-of-life issues, it had nothing to do with shifting his career focus. He does not dwell on the past. He does not use terms like 'in my day.' He feels he did the right thing by leaving the stem cell field when he was at the top of his game.

He was quick to see the potential – negative and positive – of the Internet. In 1996 he co-authored a paper with Musa Mayer, an American breast cancer survivor and cancer patient advocate, on the impact of the Internet on people living with cancer.[37] He became an early advocate of providing public access to peer-reviewed medical research reports via the Web, chairing a national task force whose work led directly to the creation, in 2007, of an open access policy by the Canadian Institutes of Health Research. He edits one blog on the open access movement and another on cancer stem cells.

McCulloch, in direct contrast, stayed busy with blood. Sutcliffe describes him as 'a consummate biomedical scientist' who was focused on inquiring 'into a very discrete area, hematological malignancies.' So he built a total career focus on stem cells. 'Bun was a driven person. He clearly had a passion. He had a belief in what he was doing and of what needed to be done. It was totally a passion that was driven by hematopoietic research that could drive the decisions in clinical leukemia. Bun wasn't really looking to get outside of that and become more involved in other types of science and biology.'

McCulloch suggested that Till's success in areas other than stem cell science illustrated a range of interests that he himself lacked. 'Jim moved from being a physicist to become a biologist, and then he moved even further and became a sociologist. He's interested intellectually in measurements of the quality of life and issues of that sort. I'm still an experimental hematologist, if you like. I have – intellectually and professionally – moved very little.'

Ron Worton, the Canadian scientist who in 1986 identified the dystrophin gene responsible for Duchenne muscular dystrophy, did his PhD at the OCI in the 1960s. McCulloch, he says, intimidated him so much that he shied away from much one-to-one contact, until he needed help with a paper.

'I had written my first paper. I knew it was a bit long and it was a bit pedantic. I went to show it to McCulloch. I gave him a copy, and he said to come back and see him at nine o'clock the next morning. So I came back and he said, "Well, everything's in there and the scientific conclusions are good and I liked many aspects of it, but it's not the way I would write it. Let me tell you the way I would write it." And he picked up his Dictaphone, and for the next half hour he paced back and forth in his office with his Dictaphone in his hand, and he dictated the entire paper from front to back. And I sat there thinking, "I just spent four weeks writing this thing and redrafting it and redrafting it, and he's written a much better paper in a half an hour by speaking into his Dictaphone." So you can see why many of the students and postdocs would be a little bit intimidated to talk to him, at least in the early days of their time there.

'I realized as I was going through the paper that this was a much more exciting way to write, it was more dynamic, it was more interesting. After that, for the second part of my time there, I would talk to him often and he would have just wild ideas: "Why don't we try this experiment?" or "Why don't we do that?" And I'd go back to my space and think about it and probably more than half of his suggestions were not workable. But the fact is that there were a lot of really wonderful ideas coming out of his head that I could then think about and pick and choose what I was going to do.'

The McCulloch lessons helped Worton in his career. He went on to found the Canadian Stem Cell Network in 2001, establishing it as a model for formalizing cooperation and collaboration among scientists from the array of fields and disciplines involved in regenerative medicine. That organization, hosted by the University of Ottawa, is part of Canada's Networks of Centres of Excellence program. It channels $6.4 million in annual federal funding to almost one hundred researchers at more than fifty universities and hospitals to advance the translation of stem cell research into clinical applications and commercial products. Each year the Network honours a Canadian researcher who has made an outstanding contribution to stem cell science. It is, of course, called the Till and McCulloch Award.

5

The Progeny

Fifty years ago, Jim Till and Ernest McCulloch were hard at work in their lab at the Ontario Cancer Institute in Toronto trying to solve the riddle of bone marrow to find out how the body makes blood and how cells repopulate and replenish. Today, Guy Sauvageau, CEO and Scientific Director of the Institute for Research in Immunology and Cancer in Montreal, is trying to find ways to make bone marrow repopulate and replenish blood cells better.

The times have changed, the quest has not. What drove Till and McCulloch to make their scientific discoveries now drives Sauvageau. 'I've always been fascinated by the microscope, by the studies of blood cells, he says. 'That's why I went into hematology. Leukemia was always of interest, and then stem cells. Connie Eaves has been a major figure in my training, in the rigour of the assays that she learned with Till and McCulloch. So, we all nucleate from that initial group and from those important discoveries.'

There are hundreds of health researchers in the field of regenerative medicine in labs across Canada and around the world who, in ways large and small, directly or indirectly, nucleate from Till and McCulloch. They are the progeny, replicating what Till and McCulloch did, differentiating it into new solutions for old problems. Some, like Connie Eaves, worked directly with the two fathers of stem cell science and have carried on, broadening its impact. Others, like Sauvageau, worked with someone who worked with them. And so on and so on as the work done a half-century ago gets carried forward.

To put it another way: Till and McCulloch figured out how the first key pieces fit together in the gigantic jigsaw puzzle that is stem cell science. Others have since added, and continue to add, connecting pieces.

The big picture, however, is still far from clear. Old frustrations, such as the early failures in bone marrow transplantation, have given way to new ones, such as the inability to do more transplants for more people.

'Even today, I would say 10 per cent of the patients who go for an autologous transplant [one using their own bone marrow cells] will not get a transplantation,' says Sauvageau. 'We cannot mobilize a sufficiently high number of stem cells from their marrow to transplant them. In terms of the allogenic transplants, those receiving cells from a donor, I would say this number is probably close to 30 per cent – again because of this issue.'

To Sauvageau, Till and McCulloch are heroes. He remembers coming down with a case of the nerves when he met them at a conference. 'It was a mixture of pride and being nervous at meeting people that you've read about. There's an aura that surrounds them.'

But if his nerves failed him, his nerve has not: he has taken their work much further. In 2003 he published a breakthrough paper in *Nature* implicating a gene called Bmi-1 as a tumour generator in leukemia and identifying another, HoxB4, as key to stem cell proliferation.[38] In a 2009 paper in *Cell* he demonstrated how to scale up large volumes of stem cells from a small number of bone marrow cells. The finding could have impacts in making bone marrow transplantation more accessible to more people who need it.[39]

Much like McCulloch was, he is fascinated by the secrets of stem cell proliferation. 'One of the most difficult aspects of chemotherapy is the fact that you deplete people's endogenous stem cell populations. If we had a factor that enhances stem cell expansion while people are receiving chemotherapy, then their marrow would be protected from the secondary effects – these nasty secondary effects.' The result, Sauvageau says, would be that cancer patients get the benefit of the full dose of chemotherapy without being put into a terribly weakened state. He believes it can be done. 'We now have cells that we put into conditioned media and they expand, so we know that there's a protein or something in the conditioned media which drives their proliferation and expansion. We're working very hard on characterizing this.'

Neural, Retinal, and Pancreatic Stem Cells

If the pursuit of new knowledge by Sauvageau and other Till and McCulloch progeny is dogged, the speed at which it occurs can be frustratingly slow. Many scientists have toiled for years in search of a tiny piece that might fit into the larger puzzle. More often than not they find parts that don't fit and test hypotheses that prove to be false. In the truest sense, scientific research – especially stem cell research – is a trial-and-error occupation.

But sometimes serendipity steps in. To an extent, Till and McCulloch got lucky. They were testing for radiation sensitivity when they happened on their 'colony-forming units.' Samuel Weiss was similarly fortunate. He was doing something else entirely when he discovered that the brain has cells that can help it repair itself – neural stem cells. The publication of his findings, titled 'Generation of Neurons and Astrocytes from Isolated Cells of the Adult Mammalian Central Nervous System,' in *Science* in 1992[40] snapped into place another important piece of the stem cell jigsaw puzzle.

'It was a good experiment gone bad,' says Weiss, Director of the Hotchkiss Brain Institute in Calgary. 'It really had nothing to do with neural stem cells; it had to do with using epidermal growth factor in an attempt to keep embryonic mouse neurons alive. The neurons all died. But over time, as the neurons were dying, something else was growing in the Petri dish, and it turned out what was growing were neural stem cells that were beginning to divide in response to the growth factor. It was not the experiment that we intended. It was a complete accident.'

Timing also helped. The myth that emerged about the discovery holds that the specimen had been left unchecked while someone was on holiday, inadvertently allowing enough time for the stem cells to start proliferating. Not quite, says Weiss. 'It was something that normally you would have ignored and thrown it out. But it just so happens that somebody took a look at it later than we normally would have looked at it.'

Calling it luck doesn't do justice to the amount of work that Weiss and his colleagues had to put into analysing exactly what was going on with the cells to prove that they were, in fact, stem cells. Just as McCulloch had the intellectual curiosity to carry on investigating the bumps he found on his mouse spleens that Sunday in 1960, Weiss had the smarts to follow up on what he found was growing in the Petri dish. 'It's an important lesson,' says Weiss, 'about keeping your mind and your eyes wide open when you are doing the research and looking for the unexpected.'

Weiss also candidly admits that his investigations into neural stem cells borrowed heavily from assays designed for blood-based stem cells thirty years earlier. 'We looked at hematopoietic stem cells as a guide,' says Weiss. 'I went and took a hard look at that literature and it led back to work of Till and McCulloch.'

His discovery of neural stem cells led him to further inquiries, such as investigations into prolactin – a hormone that promotes lactation in pregnant women – as a possible treatment for multiple sclerosis. Again, keeping his eyes open helped: he began the research after noticing that women with MS tend to go into remission during pregnancy when their prolactin levels spike. 'All of the experiments we've done in animals have continued to bear fruit, so now it's time to see whether or not this can show some benefit to patients.'

A major achievement Weiss does not get credit for in the scientific literature is bringing Derek van der Kooy into the fold of stem cell science 'from the side,' as van der Kooy describes it, after a chance meeting in a bar at a conference in New Orleans.

'I mentioned we were studying these cells in the lining of the ventricles that were proliferating in the adult brain,' says van der Kooy, a Professor in the Department of Molecular Genetics at the University of Toronto, 'and he was saying they just had a new finding, it wasn't published yet, that was going to come out in *Science.* They had isolated the cells that looked to be neural stem cells from somewhere in the adult brain. We both said, "Gee, I wonder if we're both studying the same population of cells?"' That chance meeting led to a collaboration that resulted in what van der Kooy calls 'three more really good papers,' including one in *Neuron* in 1994 in which 'we just stole the techniques that the blood stem cell people had used to characterize the blood cell and used [them] as the main techniques to study neural stem cells.'

Van der Kooy agrees with Weiss that the work they did in neural stem cells was greatly assisted by what Till and McCulloch had already done. 'We were following the same paths they had already blazed, in a new tissue. So it was really useful to know the techniques they'd used to try to characterize blood stem cells because we were using similar techniques to try to characterize them in the brain.'

While most researchers tend to hone in on one area of investigation, making it their life's work, van der Kooy goes where his curiosity leads. In 2000, his lab was the first to isolate adult mouse retinal stem cells, publishing the findings in *Science.* In 2004, his lab was the first to isolate human retinal stem cells. That same year his lab identified individual cells in the adult mouse pancreas capable of making insulin-producing beta cells.

Van der Kooy hopes to find possible stem cell-derived treatments for blindness caused by retinitis pigmentosa. His original experiments have shown potential, with small improvements in vision in the mice transplanted with human photoreceptors. He thinks he can do better. 'Most recently, we've been putting our transplanted retinal cells into a hydrogel, which is something that was developed by [the University of Toronto's] Molly Shoichet, and it will distribute the cells in a nice thin layer across the entire surface of the retina. Initially, when we put our cells in, they all clumped up together in one place in the eye and so that really limited the number of cells we could integrate.'

His lab is also investigating the potential use of insulin-positive pancreatic stem cells to treat diabetes. He's still in early stages, conducting experiments with mice, but 'it seems to be working.'

The Cancer Stem Cell Discovery

Like Weiss and van der Kooy, John Dick cast back to the work of Till and McCulloch when he was making some of his ground-breaking discoveries. In 1994 he was the first to identify cancer stem cells in leukemia. Three years later, he was preparing a paper for *Nature Medicine* when he recognized that the work he was doing dealt with some of the same issues McCulloch had been wrestling with in the 1960s.

'Eventually I kind of realized, maybe it's addressing this issue of the cell of origin ... things that McCulloch had been writing about and thinking about many decades earlier. So I sent him a copy of the paper to see what he thought about it and to get some advice. He thought that the data [were] a really important demonstration of hierarchy – that acute myeloid leukemia was organized as a hierarchy. He wasn't as enamoured of our idea of the cell of origin.'

Dick, a Senior Scientist at the Toronto General and Princess Margaret Hospital Research Institutes, has championed the notion that all cancer cells are not created equal, that in some cases a rare number of them possess stem cell qualities and are actually responsible for continuously sparking the production of tumours. Essentially, he has changed how scientists think about cancer. His work has led to widespread investigations to determine whether it is these cancer stem cells that must be eliminated to keep cancer from coming back after chemotherapy and surgery have done their work on the regular tumour cells. Because cancer stem cells don't succumb to those long-established therapies, novel drugs are needed to complement the current cancer care regimes.

Like Till and McCulloch, whose 1961 paper did not immediately set the scientific world on fire, Dick did not get a great reaction straight away after his startling take on how cancer is created and maintained. He has described the research community's reaction to it as 'benign neglect.'[41] Researchers apparently felt that the findings applied only to blood-based cancers, not solid tumours. But subsequent publications – including his and other researchers' follow-up discoveries of cancer stem cells at work in solid tumours in the brain, breast, and colon – have given the cancer stem cell theory significant credence and made it perhaps the most exciting area of cancer research in the twenty-first century.

It is still a hotly debated theory (see Chapter 7), with other researchers arguing about how rare cancer stem cells are in various forms of the disease. Controversy, however, has fazed Dick no more than it did McCulloch. He has faith in the power of asking the right research questions – and in building on work that others have done. In 2008, he published an article in the journal *Blood* that laid out the historical underpinnings of the cancer stem cell field, reaching back as far as the late 1800s to prove that the notion that tumours contain some cells that are more potent than others is actually an old one that was rediscovered and proven with new technology.[42]

'You should always look at the history when you're guiding your current experiments,' he says, 'so that you don't end up reinventing the wheel.' In that regard, the 1960s-era papers by Till and McCulloch were important to his work in identifying cancer stem cells. 'All the principles that we worked on, all the principles that our work provided more conclusive evidence for, had all been predicted by their earlier work and the work of others that had gone on in the 1950s.'

A direct research descendant of Till and McCulloch, Dick began his postdoctoral training in 1984 at the Ontario Cancer Institute, where he first met two of the key influences on his career. 'My mentors definitely are Alan Bernstein and Bob Phillips. Alan had one of the leading labs, or early labs, that got into using viruses – retroviruses – to transfer genes. Bob played a huge role in understanding stem cell function that sort of emanated right after Till and McCulloch. A lot of the principles they had initially developed, Bob ended up taking to the next level.'

In fact, Dick has a double connection: 'I did my PhD with Jim Wright in Winnipeg and Jim was a postdoc at the OCI in the early 1970s.'

Almost as important as his cancer stem cell research is the feat Dick accomplished in establishing an internationally accepted model for conducting blood research. He developed an assay for studying the repopulation of human blood stem cells in an immune-deficient mouse. It has become the standard for investigating leukemia and other blood-borne diseases. And his cancer breakthroughs have continued through the years: in 2006, he identified a population of human colon cancer stem cells that can initiate tumour growth.[43]

Much like McCulloch several decades ago, Dick is focused on identifying leukemia stem cells and developing therapies to target them to prevent cancer from recurring. He is co-leader of a multi-year, multimillion-dollar Californian/Canadian project to test novel drugs for treating leukemia. He has made inroads into identifying normal human hematopoietic stem cells and all the downstream progenitors that, together, make up the roadmap of human blood development.

West Coast Transplantation

For Connie Eaves, who has co-authored more than 250 peer-reviewed papers in a career that spans forty years, it all started at the OCI.

The Vice-President of Research at the BC Cancer Agency and Senior Scientist at Vancouver's Terry Fox Laboratory, Eaves remembers showing up for work on Sherbourne Street in 1970 on her return to Canada after completing her PhD in the United Kingdom.

'I was seven months pregnant, which wasn't a big deal for me. But I think it took Bunny and Jim by surprise because I hadn't written them about it. Initially I had communicated with Bunny. I basically arrived and walked in the door of the office, and he took one look at me and said, "Let's go up and talk to Jim." And the next thing I knew, Jim was going to be looking after me. I don't know whether it was because I was female or because I was pregnant or [because] he felt that I would be better supervised by Jim as my immediate person or what.

'But I worked with both of them quite closely the whole time I was there. And, you know, I would go down and sit in Bun's office and talk to him in the afternoon quite frequently. I mean, the only thing I really cared about was that I was given respect for my academic ability and my research ability, and I always felt I had that from both Jim and Bun from the get-go.'

Eaves did three years of postdoctoral work at the OCI. Then, as one of her colleagues described it, she 'took it all out to the West Coast.' In effect, she transplanted the OCI approach to conducting stem cell science. 'One of the things that Jim and Bun absolutely embodied was a complete and unquestioned devotion to truth. So there was never, ever, any kind of doing anything because it would gain prestige or kudos if it meant somehow twisting the truth in some way. Or that it would be transient, and the truth would come out later. They gathered around them people who wanted and liked to identify with those kind of morals. One of the reasons that they're very proud of the community is because it perpetuates that sort of philosophy and integrity.

'That's not to say that they weren't clever about how to present information – because how you market information is very important to having it understood and recognized. But that's completely different from the many ways that science is introduced and presented, based on the assumption that it doesn't matter so much if it's really true because it'll all come out in the wash, or this will be the jumping point to something else. "The end is more important than the means" or whatever that phrase is. There was never any of that.'

Some of Eaves's more notable achievements have come in recent years. Working with Australian researchers, her lab isolated stem cells from breast tissue that could regenerate milk-producing mammary glands in mice – a first in the field of stem cell science. The results were published in *Nature* in 2006.[44] In 2007, her lab proved that adult blood-based stem cells, previously thought to be identical, have four subsets – a finding that could have profound implications for improving bone marrow transplantation.

She is investigating the root causes of cancer by expanding the understanding of the characterization and regulation of stem cells in leukemia and breast cancer. 'One of my students has discovered the pathway that causes fetal blood stem cells to switch shortly after birth to an adult program, and a postdoc is investigating whether this helps dictate the different kinds of leukemia that are seen in babies as compared to adults. Our work over the last few years in leukemia has become an even bigger group effort. It's focused on trying to understand why chronic myeloid leukemia stem cells are generally resistant to all known therapies and the use of this information to predict which patients will not respond to [the anti-cancer drug] Gleevec so they can be immediately transferred to something better – and to also search for drugs that will kill the stem cells.'

Like Till and McCulloch, Eaves has made recruiting and training the next generations of stem cell scientists a priority. Many who moved through her lab, such as Keith Humphries, an expert in the characterization of genes involved in stem cells' ability to self-renew and differentiate, and Peter Zandstra, an innovator in generating functional tissue from stem cells, have become respected leaders themselves. Encouraging young scientists is just part of the deal, says Eaves. 'Having graduate students and postdocs is to a scientist what having children is to a parent. Most creative scientists have an urge to have people that they can share their ideas with and have some role in helping to mould their thinking and give them opportunities to think new things. And then have them introduce new developments.'

Throughout the highs and lows of research, Eaves has retained a trait she learned at the OCI: the ability to keep perspective when things go wrong. 'Research is an awful thing, you know – it's just failure all the time. So if you don't have a strong sense of humour, you can't survive it. But I do really love the research life and all the wonderful returns it offers in spite of the high failure rate inevitably associated with tackling important questions.'

Toronto Looks Outward

Janet Rossant says that Till and McCulloch were 'my scientific heroes, from a long way away, before I even came to Canada.'

In 1977, Rossant, a PhD from Cambridge with postdoctoral experience at Oxford, took a one-year sabbatical replacement position at Brock University. What was an overqualified young scientist doing, taking a fill-in spot at a small Canadian university not known for its research? Love had a lot to do with it. 'I married a Canadian who I met when I was a graduate student in Cambridge,' says Rossant. 'So I moved to Canada. There just weren't a lot of jobs, or they were all filled by previous generations.'

She took the temporary Brock position and ran with it. 'I managed to argue it into a tenured position and built quite a good program there, because I was also able to collaborate and interact with people in Buffalo, at Roswell Park Cancer Institute, and people at McMaster University.'

A failed attempt to land a job at the University of Toronto brought her into contact with Alan Bernstein, the Till acolyte who had moved on to the Samuel Lunenfeld Research Institute of Mount Sinai Hospital. 'I had applied for a position in Toronto in physiology. I came and gave a seminar, and I didn't get the job. Alan was in the audience and introduced himself afterwards. At that point, as now, I was very interested in early mouse development and I was starting to use the early embryos as a means of genetic manipulation. Alan was working on retroviruses and interested to see if he could use retroviruses to genetically alter mouse embryos. So he had the retroviruses, we had the embryos, and he was interested in collaborating.'

After arriving at the Lunenfeld Institute in 1985, Rossant established a reputation for advancing the understanding of the role that genes play in embryo development. Her work with Bernstein at Mount Sinai furthered the transplantation of stem cell science in Canada beyond the original Sherbourne Street hub.

'Alan recruited people from outside and brought new things into the mix. That was important at that time and it really set the tone for growth of Toronto science over the next twenty years, building on enormous strength at places like the OCI. All of a sudden, Toronto became a lot more outward-looking and brought people from all over the world to really move science forward in exciting ways.'

Rossant left the Samuel Lunenfeld Research Institute, where she was Acting Director, in 2005 to lead research at Toronto's Sick Kids Hospital. Her lab is researching the genetic underpinning of early lineage development in the mouse embryo in order to improve understanding of embryo growth. Indicative of her stature, Rossant was a member of the global team that drew up the ethics guidelines for conducting embryonic stem cell research for the International Society for Stem Cell Research in 2007.[45]

iPS Advances

It was Rossant who encouraged talented Hungarian scientist Andras Nagy to make Canada his home, carrying the Till and McCulloch lineage further. Nagy came to the Samuel Lunenfeld Research Institute in 1989 as a visiting scientist, worked closely with Rossant, and never left.

An innovator in the field of embryonic stem cells, Nagy and colleagues made headlines in the early 1990s by growing a whole mouse from an embryonic mouse stem cell.[46] In 2005, his lab established the first two Canadian human embryonic cell lines, allowing researchers to broaden their investigations and thereby hasten scientific progress.[47] Then, in 2009, Nagy made a major contribution to Shinya Yamanaka's 2007 discovery that human adult stem cells can be reprogrammed to create new versions – induced pluripotent stem (iPS) cells – that have all the pluripotent power of embryonic stem cells. However, Japan's Yamanaka used viruses to introduce four genes into the reprogramming process. Because viruses can mix with a cell's DNA, such a process introduces the risk of causing mutations of other genes and triggering disease. Nagy's lab, working with a Japanese researcher in Edinburgh, came up with a solution – essentially a non-viral way of creating the cells and removing the four transgenes (the reprogramming factors) from the cells after they have generated stem cells.

A significant breakthrough, it remains a work in progress. 'More than half of my lab now is working on the reprogramming problems involved in the biology of these cells,' says Nagy. 'It's very, very promising – no question – for future stem-cell-based therapies. But we still are at the stage where we don't know these cells well enough. We still have to do quite a bit of basic research to make sure that these cells are going to be equivalent in all respects to embryonic stem cells, which are the gold standard for pluripotency.'

The iPS work is going on all over the globe. 'We have a collaboration with Shinya Yamanaka. We have a large international program aiming to understand the process of reprogramming. There are laboratories from Europe, the United States, and Japan involved. My lab is coordinating this whole operation.'

What fascinates Nagy is the possibility that adult stem cells could be reprogrammed to 'other destinations' than total pluripotency for potential therapeutic use. 'If we understand the reprogramming process to pluripotency, we might also be able to learn how to drive the cells into therapeutically useful cell types, instead of going back all the way totally to pluripotency and the embryonic stem cell–like state and then coming back again and differentiating them into endothelial cells or blood cells or whatever.'

The work has pushed Nagy into the international spotlight. In 2009, he was the only Canadian selected for the *Scientific American* 10, an honour roll of those who 'demonstrated outstanding commitment to assuring that the benefits of new technologies and knowledge will accrue to humanity.' The list included United States President Barack Obama and Microsoft founder Bill Gates.[48]

In terms of Till and McCulloch lineage, Nagy is something of an adopted European nephew. He has worked closely with Rossant, who studied with Bernstein, whose PhD was supervised by Jim Till. But he arrived in Canada long after Till had quit the field and McCulloch had moved on to bone marrow transplantation and running the OCI's Biological Research Division. 'I had heard of Till and McCulloch in Hungary, where hematopoietic stem cells are studied also quite thoroughly. We had good hematologists who taught this in Hungary. I have so much appreciation, it's difficult to even express.'

Disease in a Test Tube

Like Nagy, Gordon Keller is excited about the possibilities emerging from Yamanaka's discovery that adult skin cells can be induced to return to an embryonic-like state to generate various types of cells for various types of organs and tissue.

'In our lab, I could show you human heart cells, human insulin-producing cells, human liver cells, and human blood cells, all made from the same type of stem cell.'

While his lab makes different cell types, such as pancreatic beta cells and blood cells, for investigations into growing replacement organs or tissue, he sees that as a longer-term proposition. 'Certainly that's the goal of a lot of researchers worldwide, but it's going to take time to make a functional cell that's going to integrate into the adult tissue and then behave itself.' Rather, he sees the potential for more immediate impact by using the freshly derived human cells as a testing ground for a wide array of drugs to defeat diseases.

'We could use these cells either to discover drugs or to weed out those drugs that have unexpected side effects. In other words, we'd use them for predictive drug toxicology, so that when pharmaceutical companies are developing new drugs, they will now have access to a host of human cells on which they can be tested.'

The other option, he says, is applying Yamanaka's discovery by drawing stem cells from people suffering from a disease to do research that was previously impossible. 'It's disease in a test tube. We can now make these iPS cells from people with diseases and study what is wrong with the cells. It's not going to be applicable to every disease, but for some it's going to be very, very powerful. So there are enormous opportunities and applications.'

Keller did his postdoctoral work in the early 1980s at the OCI with Bob Phillips, who had been hired by Till. While he didn't work directly with the stem cell founders, Keller has felt their influence throughout his career. 'Bob was a good mentor with a very sharp, critical mind. In fact, that can be said for most of the faculty of OCI at the time. The Till and McCulloch training was of that format.' What the OCI instilled in him, he says, is the importance of 'quantitative analysis of data. You count things. That was what Till and McCulloch brought to the table: an assay in which you could enumerate stem cells. That was huge. That quantitative approach to stem cell biology stayed with everyone who trained at the OCI.'

Best known for his work on lineage-specific differentiation of mouse and human embryonic stem cells, Keller has worked in labs in Basel, Vienna, Denver, and New York City – where, in 2005, he was named Director of the Black Family Stem Cell Institute at the Mount Sinai School of Medicine. Keller was recruited back to Canada in 2007 by Goldcorp founder Rob McEwen and his businesswoman wife Cheryl McEwen, who have invested $21 million of their own money to accelerate the development of stem cell therapies from stem cell research. His return to Canada produced almost immediate results: in 2008 his team made headlines when they published a paper in *Nature* showing that they could create beating heart tissue in a test tube from embryonic stem cells.

An influential figure in regenerative medicine, Keller served a term as President of the International Society for Stem Cell Research. With more than 3,600 members worldwide, that organization is the global voice for stem cell research. In 2010 the *Globe and Mail* named him one of twenty-five Transformational Canadians – citizens who have made a difference by immeasurably improving the lives of others.

Skin-Derived Stem Cells

Another significant piece of the stem cell jigsaw puzzle fell into place in 2001, courtesy of Freda Miller, the Alberta-raised molecular biologist who was then conducting neuroscience research at McGill University in Montreal. In the pages of *Nature Cell Biology*, Miller and colleagues described how to isolate stem cells from rodents' skin and explained how similar precursors are present in human scalp.[49]

'The discovery took on a life of its own,' says Miller, who pushed the edge of the envelope further in 2006 by demonstrating that these stem cells, which she calls skin-derived dermal precursors or SKPs, can be used to restore neural cells and to rehabilitate nervous systems damaged by disease or spinal cord injury.

Now a Senior Scientist at the Hospital for Sick Children Research Institute and a McEwen Centre investigator, Miller is working with a team of researchers in Toronto and at UBC that is reconfiguring adult stem cells as Schwann cells for transplantation. 'Schwann cells are basically what build your nerves in the periphery. It's a variation on the idea of not just putting the stem cells themselves in, but making a therapeutically useful cell type out of the stem cells and putting those in.

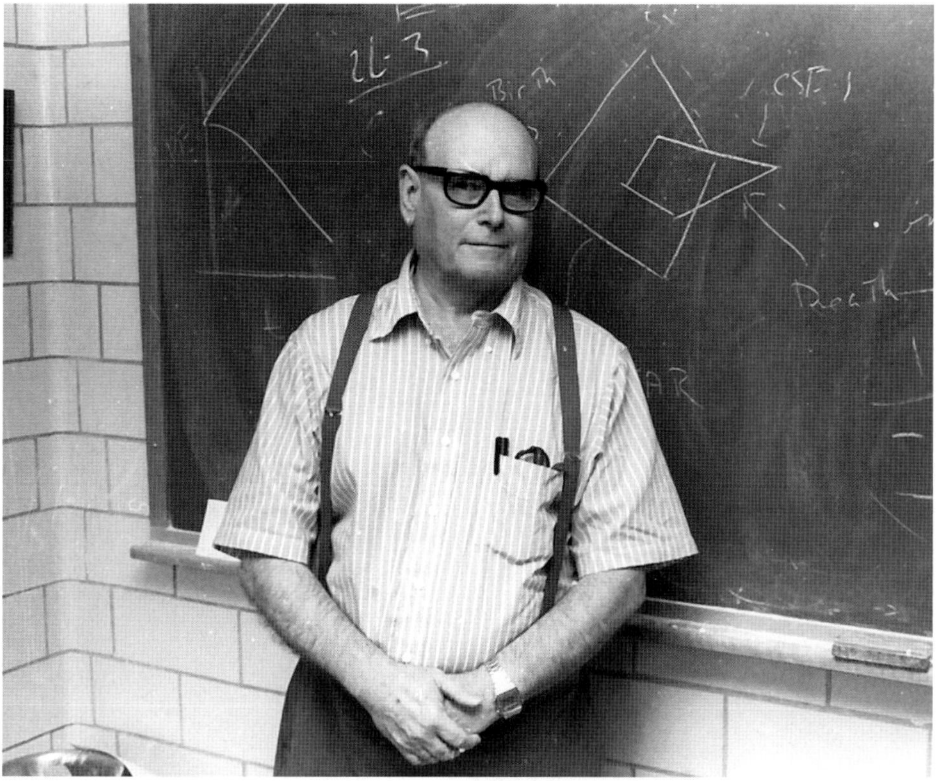

Ernest Armstrong 'Bun' McCulloch, who was fond of quoting Shakespeare and referencing Shaw, first noticed the 'spleen nodules' that proved the existence of stem cells.
(Courtesy of the University Health Network)

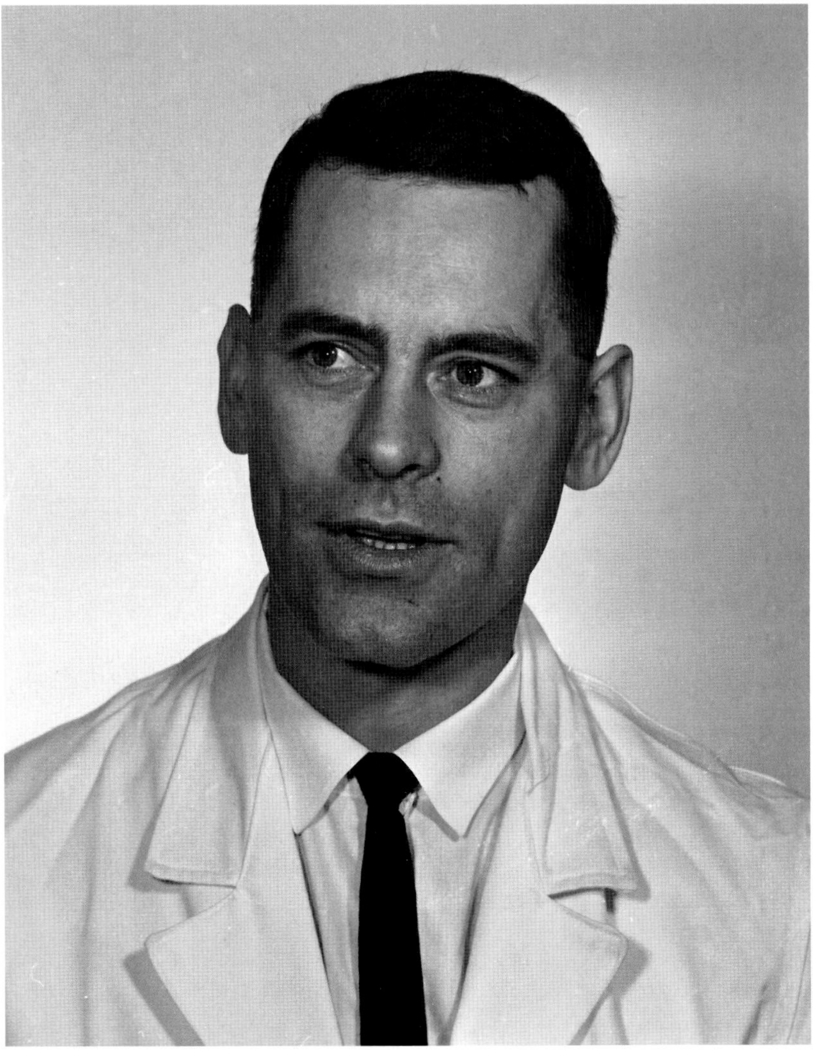

A farmboy who did time-and-motion studies in the wheat fields, James Edgar Till declined an offer from Yale to return to Canada and work at the Ontario Cancer Institute where he became McCulloch's partner.
(Courtesy of the University Health Network)

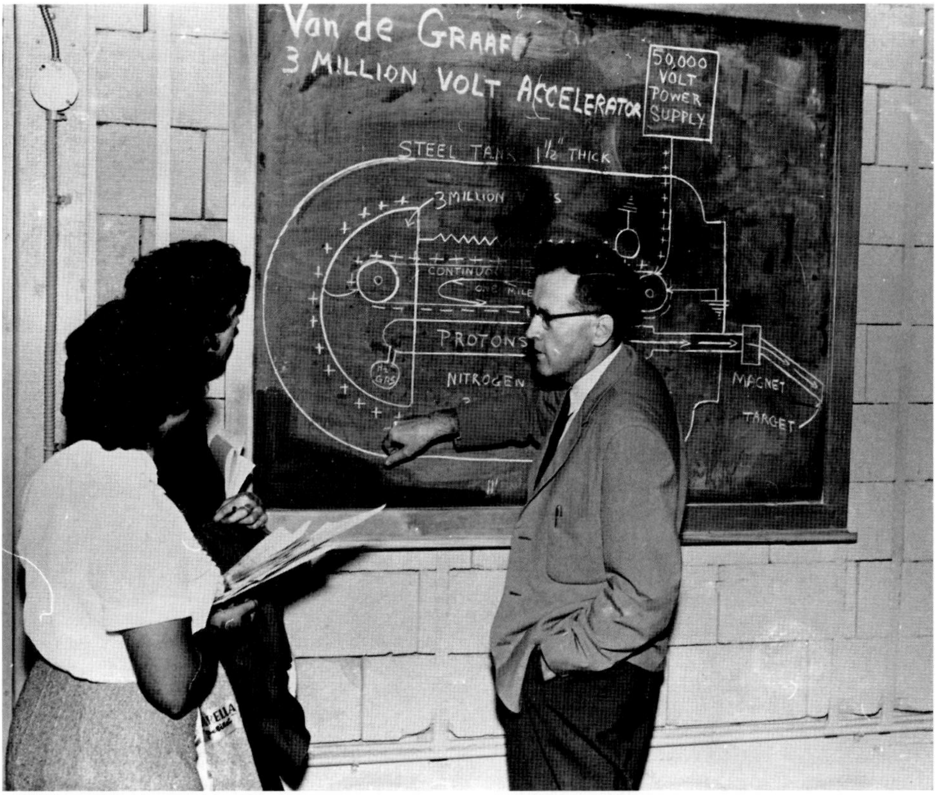

Till's mentor and boss Harold Johns pioneered the Cobalt bomb radiation treatment and demanded excellence in all things. 'He didn't put up with anything second-rate,' says Till.
(Courtesy of the University Health Network)

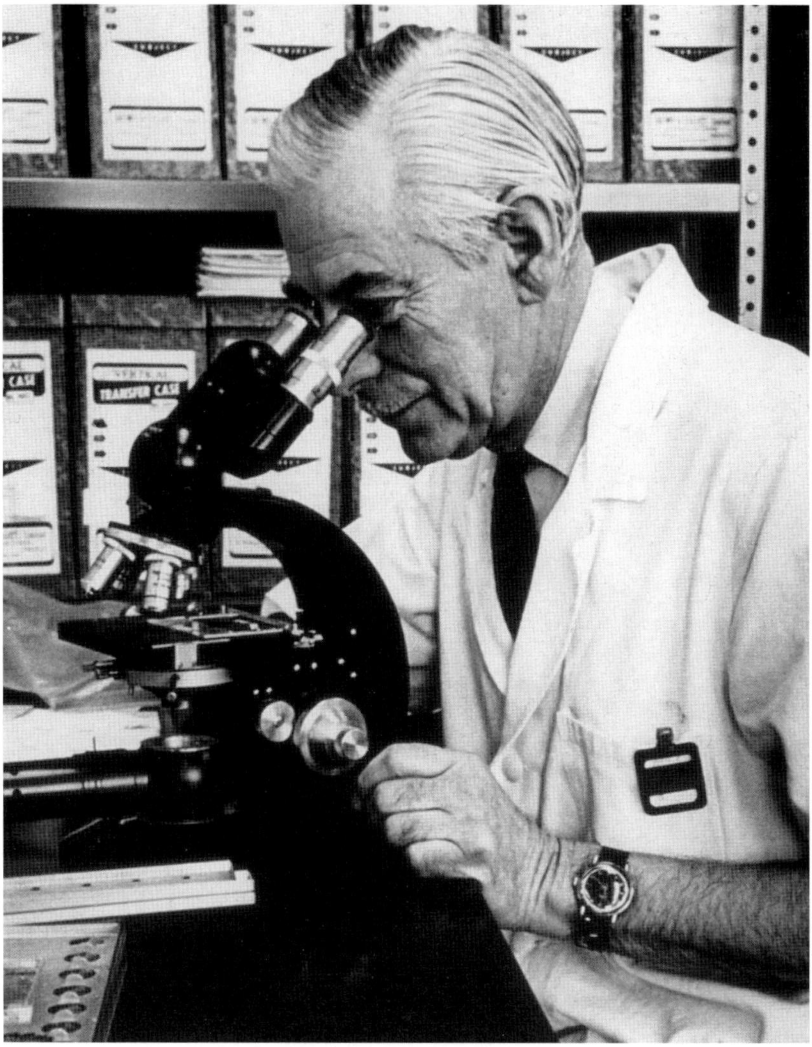

Arthur Ham, head of the Ontario Cancer Institute's Biological Research Division, hosted the gathering at which Till first heard McCulloch talk about the experiments he planned.
(Courtesy of the University Health Network)

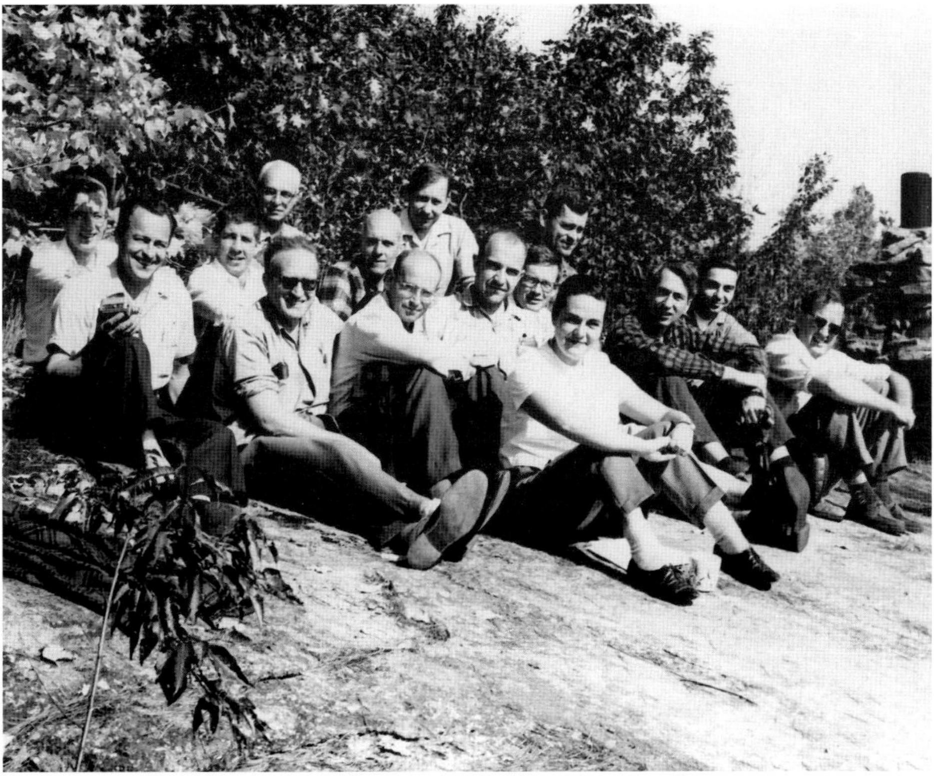

Annual retreats at rustic cottages owned by Harold Johns and his family became intellectual free-for-alls for Ontario Cancer Institute scientists. Front (left to right): Lou Siminovitch, Ernest McCulloch, Rose Sheinin, John Hunt, Arthur Axelrad, Harold Johns. Middle: Jack Cunningham, Mike Rauth, Allan Howatson, Gordon Whitmore, John Wright. Back: Clarence Fuerst (face partly in shadow), Bob Baker, Don Parsons, and Jim Till.

(Courtesy of the University Health Network)

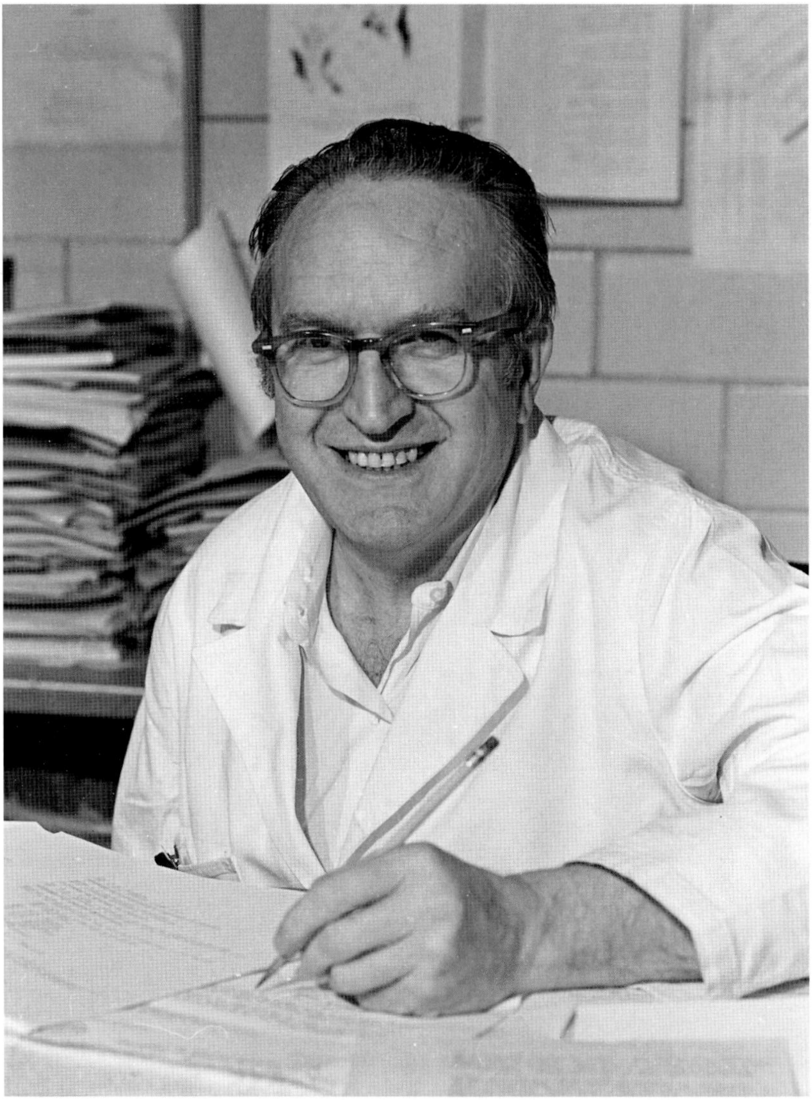

Lou Siminovitch, who partnered with Till and McCulloch on some of their most important papers, went on to create what became the University of Toronto's Department of Medical Genetics and to found the Samuel Lunenfeld Research Institute at Mount Sinai Hospital.
(Courtesy of the University Health Network)

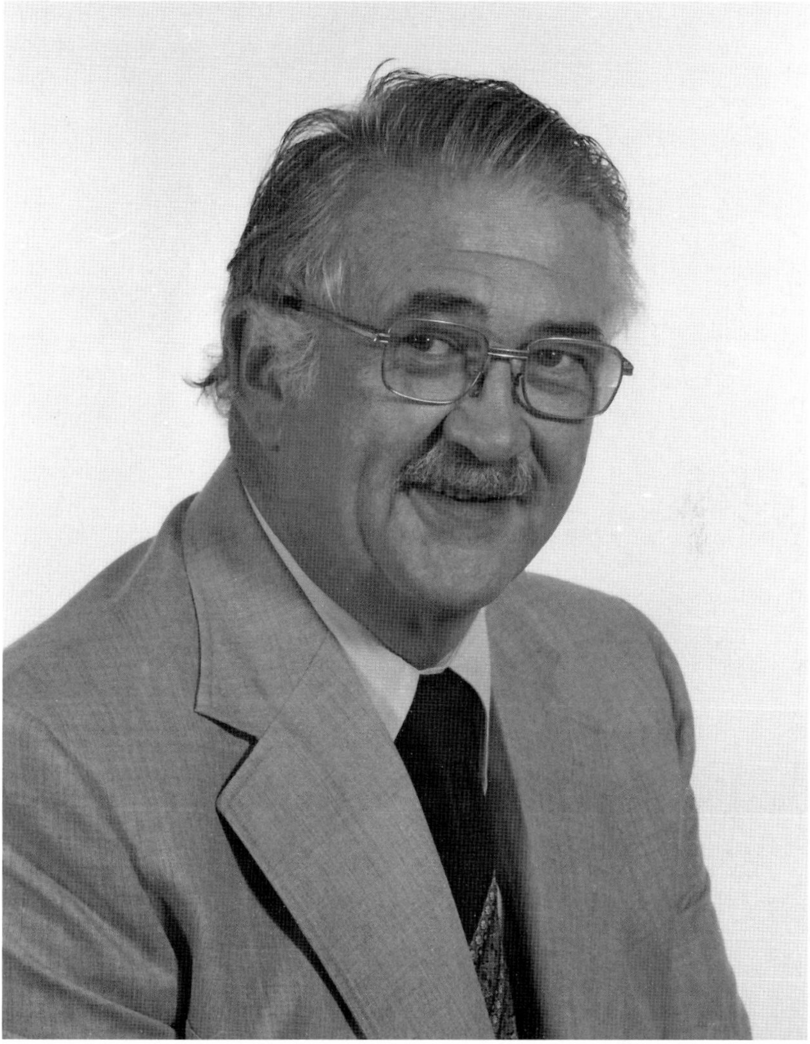

Working with McCulloch, pediatrician John Darte attempted some of the world's earliest bone marrow transplants as a treatment for leukemia in children.
(Courtesy of the University Health Network)

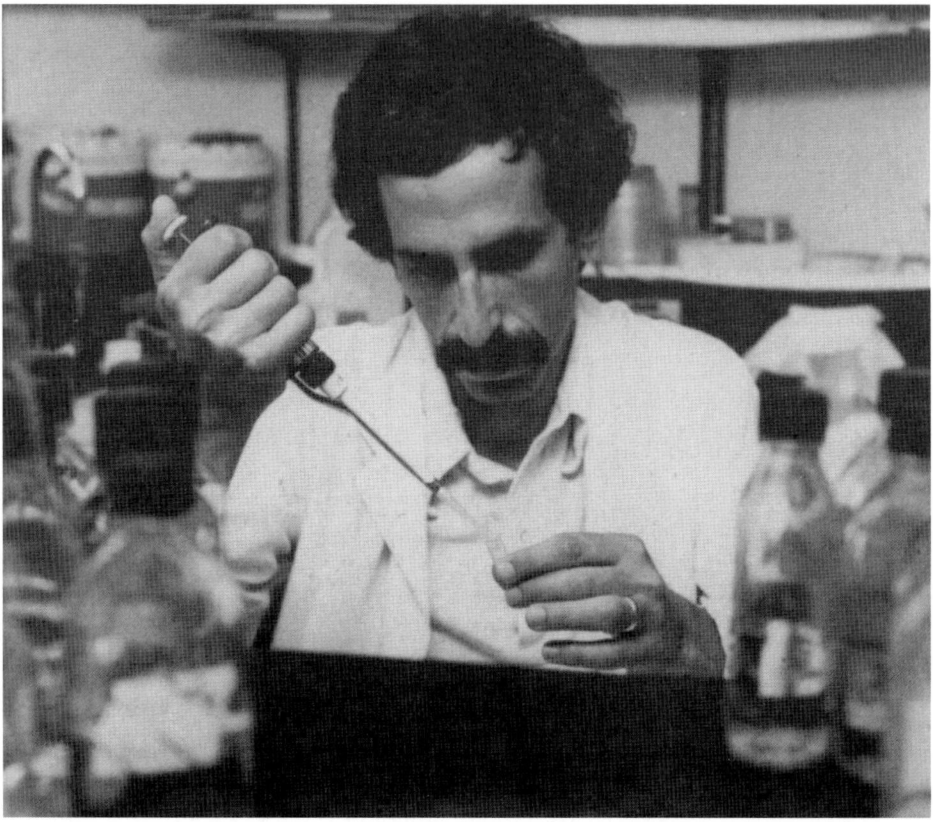

The inaugural President of the Canadian Institutes of Health Research, Alan Bernstein first toiled as a summer staffer at the Ontario Cancer Institute, and then as a PhD student with Till – whose advice he has sought ever since.
(Courtesy of the University Health Network)

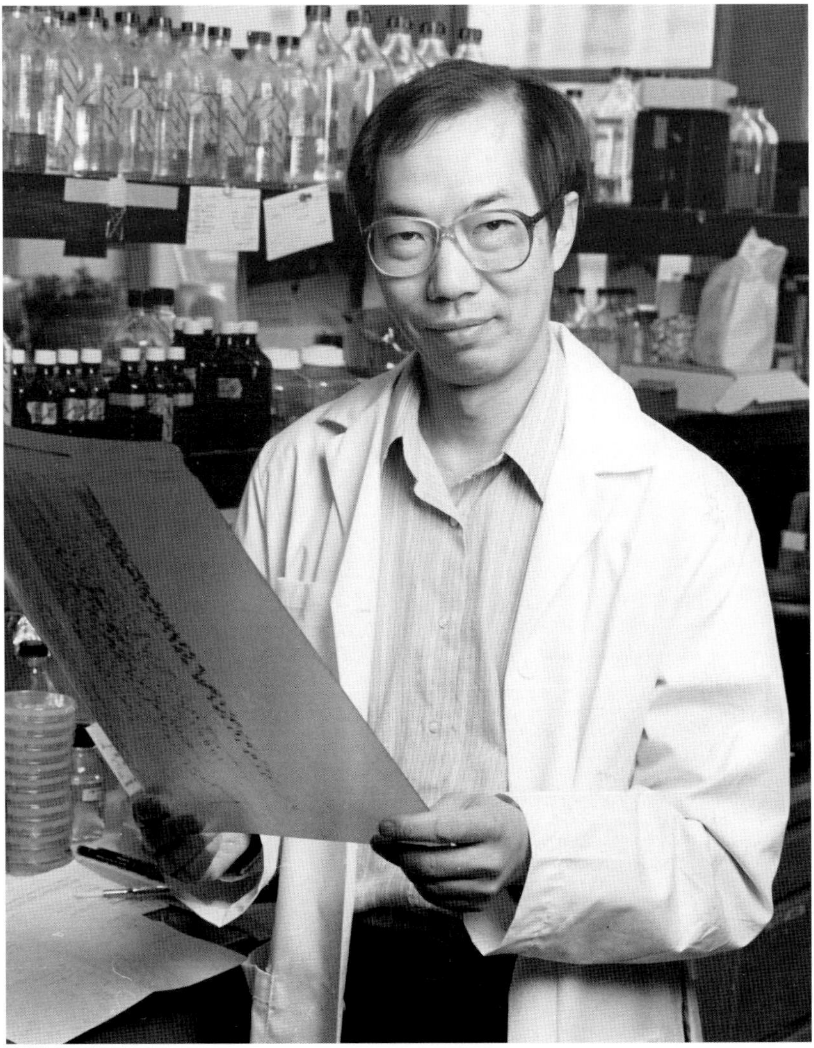

After his discovery of the T cell receptor, Tak Wah Mak rejected posts at Yale and Stanford to stay in Toronto largely out of loyalty to his mentor McCulloch. (Courtesy of the University Health Network)

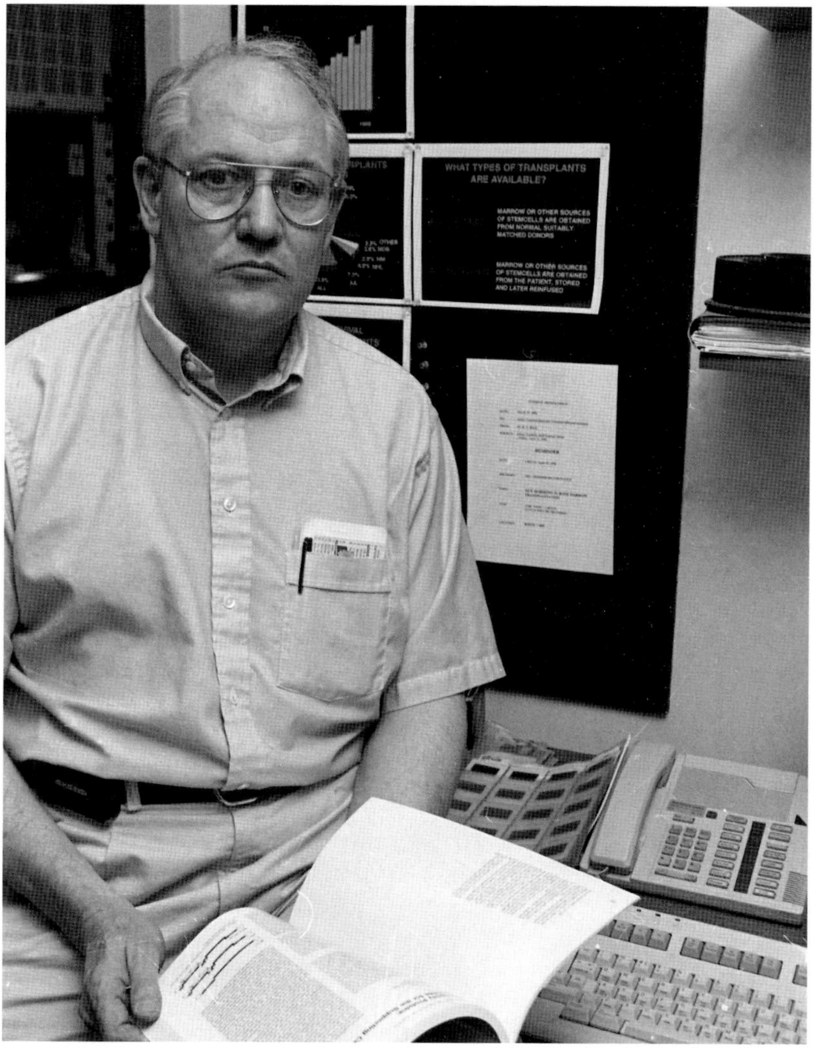

As a young medical student in Germany, Hans Messner impressed the visiting McCulloch, who told him, 'You're going to come to Toronto.' Messner went on to direct the Bone Marrow Transplant Program at the Princess Margaret Hospital.
(Courtesy of the University Health Network)

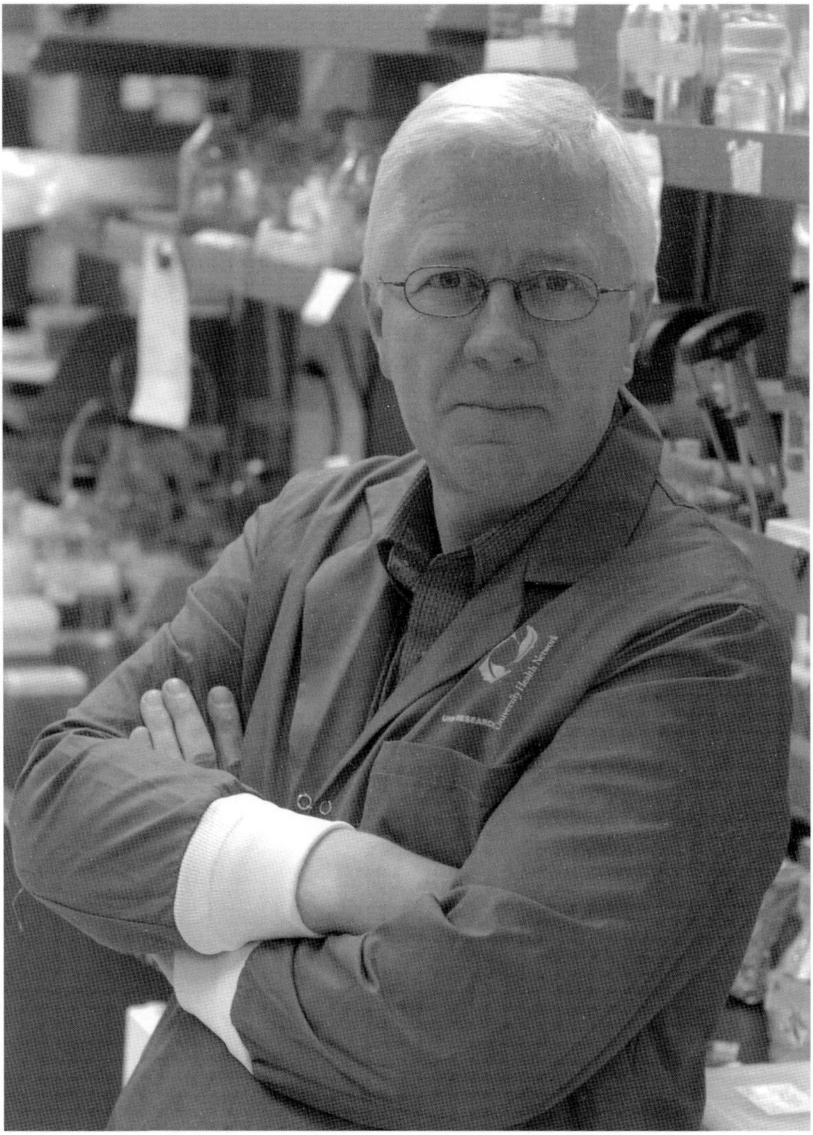

A second-generation Till and McCulloch research descendant,
John Dick identified cancer stem cells in leukemia, opening a new front
in the war on cancer.
(Courtesy of the University Health Network)

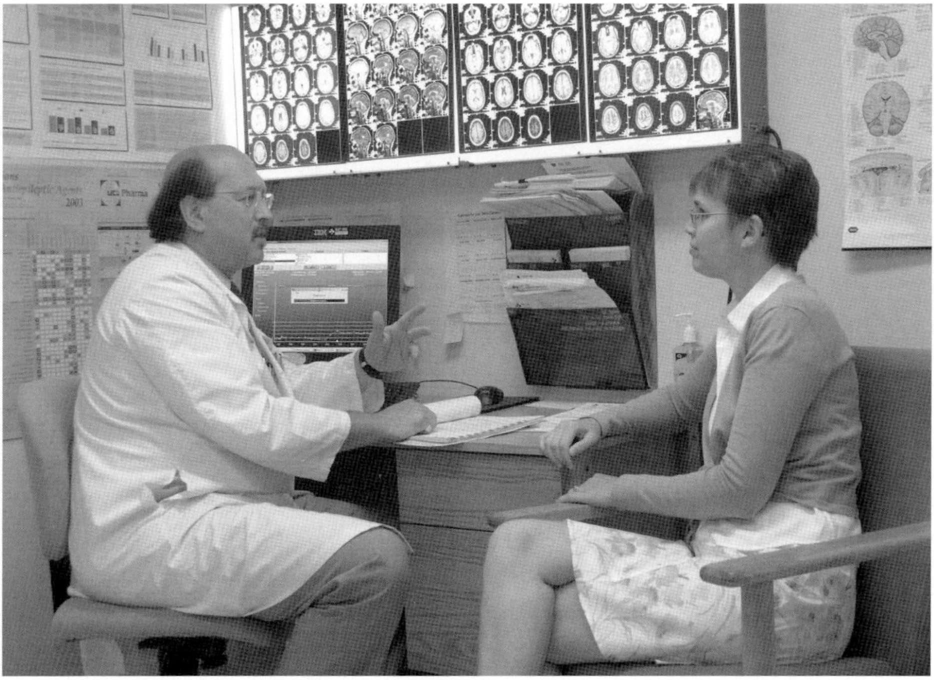

Ottawa neurologist Mark Freedman pioneered a stem cell treatment for multiple sclerosis that has given Jennifer Molson a life free from MS symptoms.
(Courtesy of Jennifer Molson)

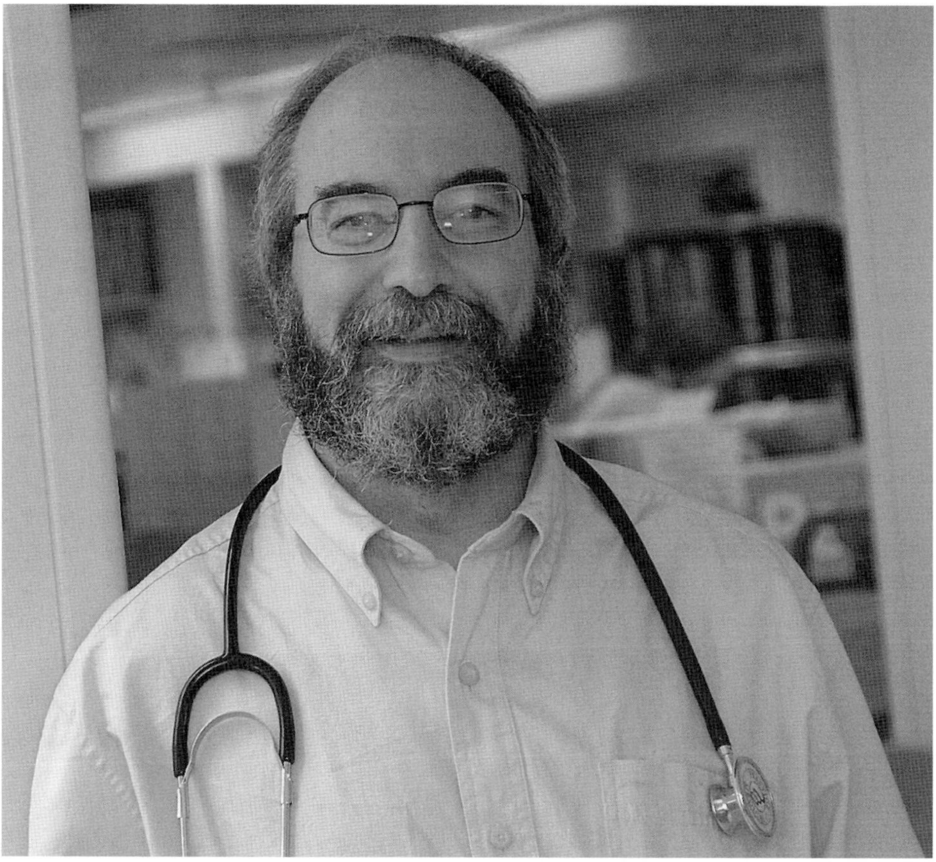

Harry Atkins, a bone marrow transplant specialist directly linked to the Till and McCulloch scientific lineage, co-leads the Ottawa MS stem cell project.
(Courtesy of the Stem Cell Network)

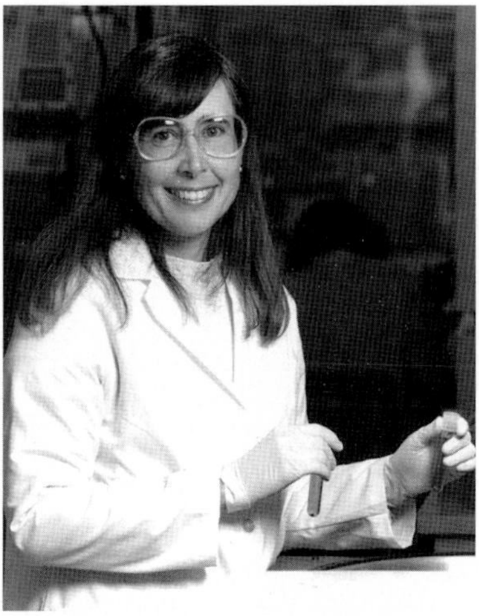

Connie Eaves, who refers to McCulloch as 'Bunny,' significantly advanced knowledge about leukemia and breast cancer after working as a Till postdoc.
(Courtesy of the Terry Fox Laboratory)

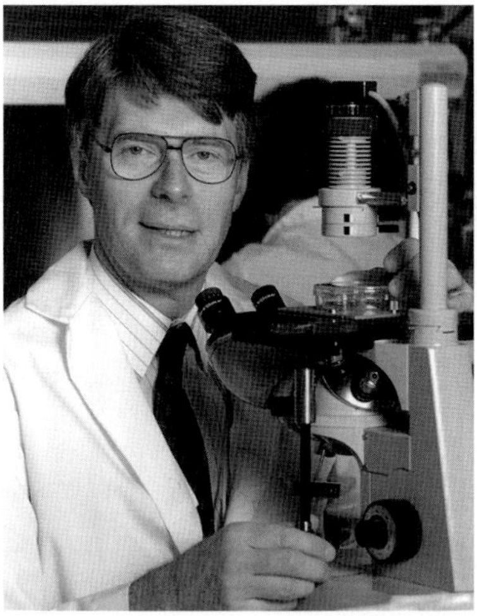

Allen Eaves, a driving force behind British Columbia's bone marrow transplantation program, says its success can be tracked back to what he learned at the Ontario Cancer Institute.
(Courtesy of the Terry Fox Laboratory)

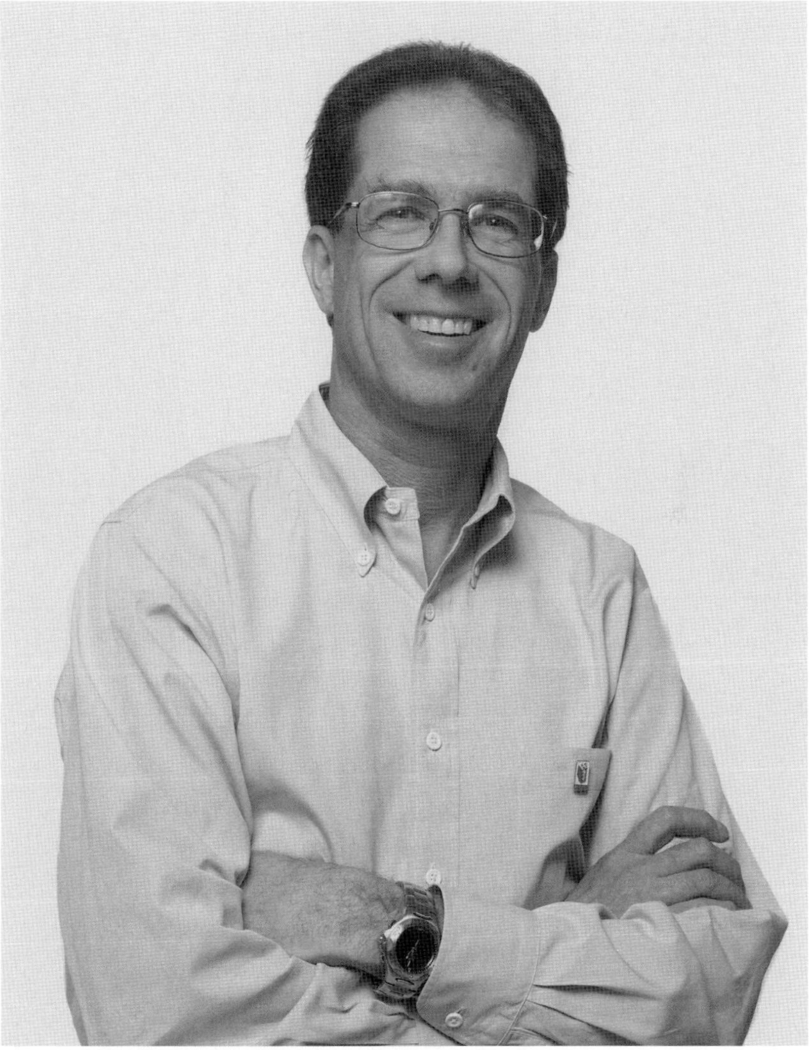

Samuel Weiss, who discovered neural stem cells, says his investigations borrowed heavily from assays that Till and McCulloch designed decades earlier.
(Courtesy of Trudie Lee)

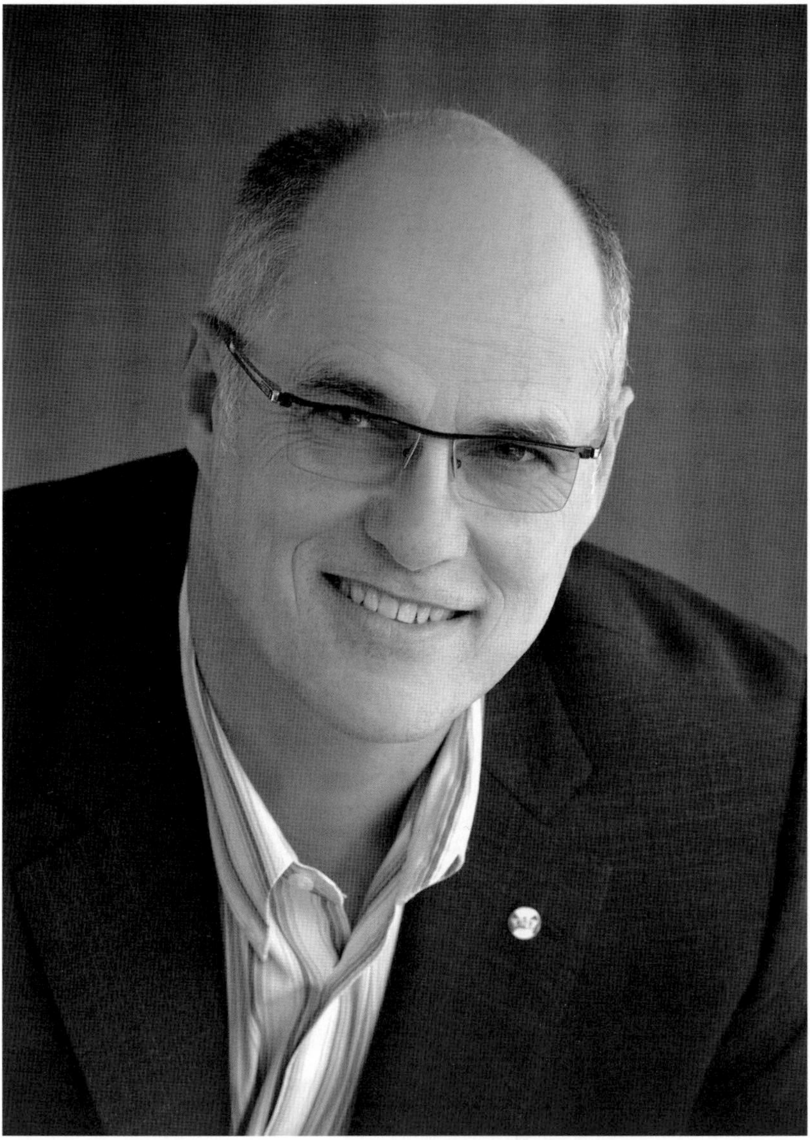

Stem Cell Network Scientific Director Michael Rudnicki has shown that tweaking stem cells that reside within us may help rebuild damaged parts. He believes 'without question' that Till and McCulloch deserve the Nobel Prize.
(Courtesy of the Stem Cell Network)

'Wolfram Tetzlaff, who is my close collaborator at the University of British Columbia, did the experiments with chronic spinal cord injury [in rodents]. Much to our surprise, it looks like it's leading to both neural and anatomical and functional recovery. We're excited about it. It validates this approach as something that might be really useful for people.'

Miller's connections to Till and McCulloch are, at best, tenuous: her influences are as much Californian as Canadian. She became a PhD at the University of Calgary and then did postdoctoral work at California's Scripps Research Institute, a private, not-for-profit organization that focuses on basic biomedical science. After becoming an Associate Professor at the University of Alberta in Edmonton in 1988, she moved on to McGill in 1993 before accepting the position at Sick Kids in 2002.

Miller's work, however, has been affected by Till and McCulloch, if only indirectly. 'Moving to Toronto and being part of the Stem Cell Network, which has so many people who are related to Till and McCulloch, has been phenomenal in terms of the development of my science. Even if my interaction with them has been more generic, certainly my conversations with their lineage have had enormous repercussions intellectually.'

If Miller's Till and McCulloch connection is more like six degrees of separation, Michael Rudnicki, Director of the Ottawa Health Research Institute's Regenerative Medicine Program, can trace his research roots right back to the OCI.

A leader in muscle stem cell biology, Rudnicki did his PhD studies at the University of Ottawa with Mike McBurney, whose own Masters and PhD studies were supervised by Gordon Whitmore at the OCI in the late 1960s and early 1970s. 'So, from the very beginning, I was thoroughly indoctrinated in the stem cell lexicon – given that McBurney worked in the shadow of Till and McCulloch.' His other connection is through Ron Worton, who recruited him to come back to Ottawa from McMaster University to take a position with the Ottawa Health Research Institute. (Worton did his PhD with Till in the 1960s.)

He admires the 'intellectual sophistication' that Till and McCulloch demonstrated in their work. 'They created the paradigm of stem cell biology. They outlined the whole intellectual framework that we're still working with today. It's quite remarkable, given that they were using very simple technical approaches. They were asking the right questions and challenging the prevailing notions.'

Rudnicki has demonstrated that a type of protein called Pax7 functions to specify the identity of muscle stem cells – a big step toward using stem cells to repair damaged or diseased tissue. His work earned him the cover of the prestigious journal *Cell* in 2000, with follow-up publications throughout the decade. His 2009 paper, published in *Cell Stem Cell*, identified a role for a secreted protein called Wnt7a in stimulating the amplification of muscle stem cells. Artificially increasing the amount of Wnt7a accelerates and augments repair of skeletal muscle.

The discoveries made by Rudnicki have helped shift the emphasis away from the notion of transplanting stem cells into tissue to make repairs toward the idea of tweaking the stem cells that reside within us to mobilize and rebuild damaged or diseased parts. His lab is focused on unravelling the molecular mechanisms at play when adult stem cells repair tissue. It is work that holds great promise for people who suffer from degenerative diseases such as muscular dystrophy, as well as those undergoing knee replacements or recovering from muscle-depleting surgery.

'We've had some discoveries that are translatable,' says Rudnicki, who succeeded Worton as Scientific Director of the Stem Cell Network. 'I'm a believer. I'm quite excited about regenerative medicine's potential to transform clinical practice, to help people we haven't been able to help before.'

One to Watch

Finally, if any further proof is needed that the work Till and McCulloch did fifty years ago will be carried forward well into the twenty-first century, it is embodied in Brad Dykstra, a young Canadian stem cell scientist now working in the Netherlands.

In 2006, when he was completing his PhD with Connie Eaves at UBC, Dykstra wrote a paper that proved something long supposed about hematopoietic stem cells but that had never actually been quantified: that some have different qualities than others. It was published in the prestigious journal *Cell Stem Cell* in August 2007 and has caused researchers to rethink the properties that stem cells pass along in their self-renewal process.

'It was beautifully done, really a technical *tour de force*,' says David Scadden, who co-directs the Harvard Stem Cell Institute and the Harvard University Department of Stem Cell and Regenerative Biology.

'It addressed an issue that many had suspected but none had defined. It's a little bit like Till and McCulloch, in a sense. The concept of a stem cell had probably been around for fifty years before they did their work and said, "This is much more than just of intellectual interest, we can actually work with it in a systematic and intelligent way." Similarly, the idea [that Dykstra and his co-authors presented] that within this population of repopulating cells there are subsets that are better at one thing than another speaks to the idea that either these cells are metastable and they can have many identities or they have different subsets that, maybe, could teach us how to do better tuning of the kind of effects we want to achieve with stem cells.'

Dykstra, who in his early thirties is still very much a fresh face in the stem cell field, is carrying on the Till and McCulloch tradition of doing paradigm-shifting work based on creative thinking and painstakingly rigorous research. It adds another piece to the puzzle – or, to use his analogy, another brick in the building.

'For me, it's great to be able to contribute to the basic understanding of one particular stem cell type, in our case hematopoietic stem cells,' says Dykstra. 'I hope that the same concepts do apply and will apply to every other stem cell out there. I'm contributing one little brick in the building that's going up all around me. I'm very proud of my brick and I know that it is important because other people are already building on it. It's gratifying, but at the same time I know it's only a brick.'

Here is the kicker: Dykstra, doing his innovative work fifty years after the pioneers did theirs, bears an uncanny resemblance to a young James Edgar Till. 'People tell me that,' he says. 'It's pretty neat.'

PART THREE

Today and Tomorrow

6

Ethics, Hope, and Hype

If politics and religion make strange bedfellows, things get even stranger when science is added to the mix.

The field of stem cell science has been marked by heated debate, so much so that simply using the term 'stem cell' is enough to upset some. Words like 'clone' also carry a weight of controversy, especially since 1996, when scientists in Scotland cloned Dolly the sheep from a single adult cell. People often forget that stem cells are used in medical practice on a daily basis. Every time a bone marrow transplant succeeds in saving a cancer patient's life, it is thanks to the hematopoietic stem cells that rebuilt the blood supply to fight off the leukemia. Cloning? In its simplest terms, it just means making a number of identical cells from a single one. The human body does it every day.

Sometimes the debate over stem cells sounds like the plot of the next Hollywood summer blockbuster. Everything from Nazis to the creation of storehouses of human 'spare parts' gets thrown into the discussion. And because the science of stem cells is itself extremely complicated, it has often been difficult to keep heated rhetoric separate from hard reality.

According to the Ontario-based website religioustolerance.org, the controversy over embryonic stem cell research 'centres on whether human life in the form of an embryo less than two weeks after conception is also a human person. If it is a person, then extracting stem cells constitutes first-degree murder. If it is not a person, then removing stem cells is morally acceptable.'[50]

For those who genuinely believe that an embryo has full moral status, this is, no doubt, a tough issue. From a research standpoint, embryonic stem cells offer the widest potential in terms of cell differentiation

– the ability to become different cells for different parts of the body. In other words, at the moment, embryonic stem cells could potentially be used for a far wider variety of medical treatments and cures than any other form of stem cell.

James Till and Ernest McCulloch never worked with human embryonic stem cells. That type of cell was not discovered until they were well past their prime years of scientific research. They were more concerned about cancer and finding a way to deploy blood-based stem cells to save lives. But because their work is so fundamental to the principles that support all stem cell science, including embryonic stem cell research, a discussion of the ethical debate in stem cell science is warranted, if for no other reason than the impact of that debate on twenty-first-century researchers who are carrying their work forward and attempting to push back the boundaries of medical science.

It is an intense debate. The passionate language used when talking about stem cells tends to get very extreme, very quickly. And it comes from people in positions of awesome authority and influence:

> Experience is already showing how a tragic coarsening of consciences accompanies the assault on innocent human life in the womb, leading to accommodation and acquiescence in the face of other related evils such as euthanasia, infanticide and, most recently, proposals for the creation for research purposes of human embryos, destined to destruction in the process.

Pope John Paul II spoke those words on 23 July 2001 to then U.S. President George W. Bush.[51] The leader of the worldwide Roman Catholic Church told the leader of the free world that embryonic stem cell research was an evil akin to the practice of killing newborn infants or old people.

The late pope's fears encapsulate one side of the debate, which began in 1998 with the discovery that scientists could obtain embryonic stem cells from early human embryos.[52] On the one hand, the breakthrough signalled the potential for using stem cells to cure disease. On the other, it immediately linked the subject of stem cells with abortion and human cloning and other hot-button, conservative-versus-liberal issues. It also heightened society's already growing anxiety about where science and technology is leading us.

Those who extract embryonic stem cells have been called murderers. In 2005, James Dobson, founder and former chairman of the American organization Focus on the Family, compared embryonic stem cell researchers to Nazis: 'In World War II, the Nazis experimented on human beings in horrible ways in the concentration camps, and I imagine, if you wanted to take the time to read about it, there would have been some discoveries there that benefited mankind. You know, if you take a utilitarian approach, that if something results in good, then it is good. But that's obviously not true.'[53]

Dobson is talking about university-supported medical researchers who are trying to find cures for Alzheimer's and Parkinson's and other degenerative diseases by working with cells derived from donated embryos left over from *in vitro* fertilization – that is, cells that have been created outside the body and donated by clinic patients who have given their informed consent. Dobson is likening these researchers to death camp fiends who severed bones from unanaesthetized prisoners. While this is a huge leap to make, it serves a purpose: to inflame an already overheated debate.

'Even if stem cell research now does not necessarily implicate embryos in the way they're often being described in popular culture, it nevertheless remains this very powerful rhetorical tool to keep the issue of the moral status of the embryo on the cultural radar,' says Timothy Caulfield, a Canada Research Chair working in Health Law and Policy with the University of Alberta.

'If you genuinely hold these views ... if you believe the embryo has full moral status – and, full disclosure, I do not – then research on it is morally reprehensible,' says Caulfield. 'But we live in a pluralistic society and if you believe the polls, if you believe the surveys, and if you believe the focus groups ... it really isn't a very large percentage of the population that holds those immutable, inflexible views of the embryo. It's been ten and fifteen percent of the population in Canada – perhaps more in the United States. The vast majority, perhaps around sixty percent, feels that an embryo has some kind of special status and deserves respect, but that if the appropriate steps are taken, if the appropriate safeguards are in place, then the benefits of science should take precedence.'

Since the 1998 discovery of embryonic stem cells, this heated ethical issue has been debated in the various governments of provinces, states, and countries worldwide. The pope's statement to President Bush threw gas on a political fire that was already blazing. Certainly, the stem cell debate found a forum in the Canadian House of Commons as well.

In 2002, after the release of a Canadian Institutes of Health Research document titled *Human Pluripotent Stem Cell Research: Guidelines for CIHR-funded Research*, the Government of Canada unveiled Bill C-56: An Act Respecting Assisted Human Reproduction, the first legislation in the country to address embryonic research. The overall purpose of the bill was to regulate assisted reproduction in Canada, but it also made a number of provisions for 'associated research.' The bill stated that licences for embryonic research could only be given for *in vitro* embryos, and 'may be issued only if the [Assisted Human Reproduction] Agency is satisfied the use of such embryos is necessary for the purpose of the proposed research.'[54] Reaction was mixed, with some seeing it as a barrier to research,[55] others as striking a balance between allowing science to advance and addressing moral issues.[56] Parliament was prorogued before Bill C-56 could be passed, but the bill was reintroduced later that year as Bill C-13: An Act Respecting Assisted Human Reproduction and Related Research. (It was later renamed C-6: Assisted Human Reproduction Act.)

During discussion of Bills C-56 and C-13 (which were essentially the same bill), many people involved in different sides of the ethical debate spoke out. According to the commentary within the bill itself:

> many witnesses, notably from the faith communities, strenuously opposed allowing research to be carried out on *in vitro* embryos. To do so, in their opinion, would be to treat such embryos as a commodity and would, in all events, result in the taking of a human life. Others expressed strong support for allowing research on *in vitro* embryos no longer required for *in vitro* fertilization (IVF) because of their potential for alleviating human suffering and disease.[57]

In a 2002 issue of *Health Law Review*, Caulfield praised the Canadian government for putting a regulatory framework for stem cell research in place, but also pointed out that the Bill C-13 prohibits certain research activities without a consensus that these activities represented a 'major social concern.'[58]

At that time, Caulfield was advocating for 'therapeutic cloning' – a term that sounds like something from a plot from a *Star Trek* episode, or from any number of sci-fi fantasies from the last half-century. But therapeutic cloning has nothing to do with creating a copy of a human being. That type of cloning, called reproductive cloning, has almost universally been deemed unethical. Therapeutic cloning refers to the ability to create a cloned embryo of a patient in order to develop stem cells that are a perfect match for them.[59] The considerable upside to this kind of therapy is that it greatly reduces the risk of rejection of implanted cells. That such cloning has yet to yield significant medical advances is beside the point, according to Caulfield. 'People say, "Oh therapeutic cloning hasn't panned out." Well that's irrelevant. Ninety-nine percent of all scientific roads that people travel down are dead ends. That's the nature of science; you can't really use that as an argument. What I'm concerned about is the nature of the banning of any area of scientific inquiry.'

In Canada and the United States, embryonic stem cells used in medical research are derived from spare eggs provided by consenting donors who underwent treatment at *in vitro* fertilization clinics – a far cry from fears of 'an assault on human life in the womb.' But that point is moot to those who believe that an embryonic stem cell – regardless of whether it's *in vitro* or *in vivo* (within a living organism) – represents a human life.

Roughly one month after the pope's 2001 statement to the American leader, President Bush addressed the American people with his own message:

> Embryonic stem cell research is at the leading edge of a series of moral hazards. The initial stem cell researcher was at first reluctant to begin his research, fearing it might be used for human cloning. Scientists have already cloned a sheep.
>
> Researchers are telling us the next step could be to clone human beings to create individual designer stem cells, essentially to grow another you, to be available in case you need another heart or lung or liver. I strongly oppose human cloning, as do most Americans. We recoil at the idea of growing human beings for spare body parts or creating life for our convenience.
>
> And while we must devote enormous energy to conquering disease, it is equally important that we pay attention to the moral concerns raised by the new frontier of human embryo stem cell research. Even the most noble ends do not justify any means.[60]

Clearly, confusion over the difference between reproductive and therapeutic cloning has affected policy making. In his address, President Bush announced that the American government would spend $250 million on research on some sixty lines of stem cells that existed at the time. However, the government would place a ban on federal funding for any lines of embryonic stem cells developed after that time.[61] This ban lasted nearly eight years, until the next president, Barack Obama, lifted it in 2009.

As this book was being written, the controversy over the use of embryonic stem cells was again raging in the United States, after a federal district court judge ruled that President Obama's executive order violated a ban on federal money being used to destroy embryos. The judge, an appointee from the Reagan era, ruled that destruction of embryos at any point in the research process constituted a breaking of the ban.[62]

Worldwide, the debate continues. Some countries, such as China, Japan, the United Kingdom, Singapore, and Belgium, have passed legislation to allow therapeutic cloning.[63] [64] Other countries' policies are more limiting. Germany does not allow the creation of embryonic stem cells for research and has only recently authorized scientists to use imported stem cell lines. Italy's policies are similarly fashioned.[65]

What are the implications of this debate for stem cell research?

Besides the fact that policies prohibiting certain forms of research can hinder work or even stop it from being done, the potential for damage could, hypothetically, be profound. When issues of medical advancement are politicized, and when information in the public domain is not readily understood, bad things can happen.

The most prominent recent example of the damage that can happen is in the domain of vaccination. In 1998, Andrew Wakefield published a paper in the British medical journal *The Lancet*. In his article, which focused on twelve children with Autism Spectrum Disorder, he suggested a link between the measles, mumps, and rubella (MMR) vaccine and the condition. Even though his data did not support his conclusion, the findings were picked up by the media and shared by concerned parents' groups, sparking a serious public backlash against MMR vaccination.

The MMR–autism debate continues to rage, even though *The Lancet* has retracted the original article, and even though a General Medical Council hearing determined that Wakefield had 'failed in his duties.'[66] Celebrities have taken sides. Former *Playboy* model Jenny McCarthy, who has become the go-to person for the media on the subject of vaccines and autism, and has written best-selling books that deal with the subject.[67] Due to the controversy, rates of MMR vaccination have fallen and rates of preventable diseases have sharply increased.[68] [69]

Another example of what can happen when science and politics collide has been various governments' responses to urgent pleas from environmentalists to accelerate action on climate change. Canada has been criticized for its reluctance to enact gas-slashing measures in the

Kyoto Protocol, and emissions continue to rise in most of the world's highly industrialized nations.

Those who doubt that man-made greenhouse gases are the true source of global warming have often called into question the science behind climate change. The sceptics' cause was bolstered in late 2009 by the 'Climategate' scandal in which stolen e-mails from the University of East Anglia's Climatic Research Unit – a key supplier of research data on climate change to the United Nations – appeared to indicate that researchers were stifling data that didn't help them make their case.

The UK scientists at the heart of the international scandal were later cleared of wrongdoing by independent investigators – though the scientists' lack of openness was criticized.[70] The damage done to the environmentalists' cause, however, was considerable, and arguments over the validity of climate change science have become even more highly charged and politicized. For example, Canada's then Environment Minister Jim Prentice had to dismiss suggestions from MP and former Cabinet colleague Maxime Bernier that he was deliberately moving very cautiously on climate change because of doubts over the scientific evidence. In a letter to a Montreal newspaper, Bernier said that the government was wise not to get tough on industry polluters: 'Every week that goes by confirms the wisdom of our Government's modest position.'[71]

The questioning of the safety of MMR vaccines and suspicions about the science behind climate change indicate a concern among some segments of society that science and scientists ought not to be trusted, that researchers have their own agenda. It is hardly surprising, then, that stem cell research presents a potential perfect storm of political controversy.

Caulfield, for one, believes that stem cell science has become a flashpoint for the broader social anxiety about where science is going and where it is leading the world. 'It's an expression of the social angst associated with science's place in our lives, with questions like "Should scientists be controlled?" and "Who are they accountable to?" and "Should we be tinkering with nature?" All those kinds of amorphous but more or less genuine concerns that you see in society. All those things are taken up in the debate around stem cell research.'

The iPS Option?

There are those who believe that the debate over the use of embryonic stem cells could soon be relegated to a side issue in regenerative medicine, overtaken by an advance that could provide an alternative source for these building-block cells. The discovery in 2007 by Japan's Shinya Yamanaka that adult cells extracted from human skin tissue can be reprogrammed back to an embryonic-like state called induced pluripotent stem (iPS) cells shocked the world of regenerative medicine. Some researchers in the stem cell community argue that iPS cells could replace the need to use embryonic stem cells, thereby throwing cold water on the heated debate.

Yamanaka, however, has stated that he worries that the iPS breakthrough may just lead back to the same argument about embryonic stem cells. 'Now, we can avoid using human embryos. So that is very good,' he told the *Toronto Star* in 2009. 'But, at the same time, we can potentially make germ cells – sperm or egg – from iPS cells. So, potentially, we can make new life from skin. That is the biggest ethical issue.'[72]

While that concern is valid; it may not be necessary to reprogram adult cells all the way back to the embryonic state. In fact, it may be more useful to transform the adult cells into later-stage progenitor cells that can be put directly to work. For example, McMaster University's Mick Bhatia has come up with a way to make progenitor blood cells out of adult skin cells, skipping the embryonic state altogether. The reprogrammed cells could be ideal for replenishing the blood supply of cancer patients who have undergone chemotherapy, while avoiding the debate over embryonic stem cells entirely.[73]

As well, many stem cell scientists have also begun to focus their efforts away from infusing or injecting embryonic stem cells into a damaged organ or tissue to fix it in favour of finding ways to mobilize the body's innate stem cells to generate repairs from within. In a 2009 magazine article, Freda Miller, the Canadian scientist credited with discovering adult stem cells in skin, put it this way: 'There are two big concepts in stem cell science right now. One is transplanting stem cells. The second is trying to get the stem cells that are there to regenerate tissue better.'[74] In Canada alone, studies are under way to test the effectiveness of using neural stem cells to stimulate the growth of neurons to replace cells damaged by stroke. Others are investigating whether it's possible to tweak proteins to regenerate muscle tissue – something that could be useful for people receiving knee or hip replacements or recovering from surgery.

For many researchers, however, embryonic stem cells remain the gold standard, the superior source material for scientific investigation. And their research results are moving ever closer to clinical application.

'I think there's some quite exciting opportunities with embryonic stem cells,' says Janet Rossant, who heads research at Toronto's Sick Kids' Hospital. 'Making retinal pigment epithelium to deal with some forms of macular degeneration – that looks like it could move to the clinic in the not-too-distant future. It's been done in the United Kingdom. And I think that in terms of diseases that could move to the clinic in the not too distant future, diabetes certainly is one. Of course, we have clinical protocols and people are close to being able to get embryonic stem cells to generate really strong insulin-producing cells, so I think that that's not so far away.'

The fact that stem cell scientists are moving closer to curing crippling diseases that have remained incurable since Hippocrates took up medicine could trigger a tipping point for social attitudes about stem cell science and the use of embryonic stem cells. It will certainly bring the debate – and the choices involved – into focus. When regenerative medicine moves beyond its current what-if state to one in which it offers evidence-based, reproducibly researched cures for devastating diseases that are killing people's parents and children, those choices will be very clear. And that time is coming.

Hope versus Hype

As the largely faith-based debate over the use of embryonic stem cells continues to simmer, controversy over those who would exploit the promise of stem cells to prey upon people has flared well beyond religious boundaries and into the public consciousness.

There is only a one-letter difference between 'hope' and 'hype.' In the world of stem cell science, those looking to cash in often transform the former into the latter. Because stem cell science offers such great hope, it is susceptible to manipulation by those who are out to profit at the expense of those whose sense of desperation is driving them to try untested and unproven experimental treatments.

The stem cell research establishment may have to shoulder at least part of the responsibility for creating this situation. In the past decade, hardly a news cycle has gone by without the trumpeting of a potential stem cell breakthrough in the fight against cancer or some other deadly or degenerative disease. While a strong case can be made for blaming the media for sensationalizing science, it often has been conventional, university-supported, fully accredited scientists who have been blowing the horns. As Lori P. Knowles explains in her article 'Stem Cell

Hype and the Dangers of Stem Cell "Tourism,"' the research world has set the bar for expectations exceptionally high:

> Stem cell researchers have walked a fine line between enthusiastically describing the long-term potential of stem-cell therapies, which helps get support for their work, and in cautioning that science and research take time and sustained support. Part of the tension for researchers lies in the need to work slowly and carefully, and yet also to attract industry funding based on the potential commercial and clinical applications from their work. Increasingly, universities and government funders are looking at commercial applications and numbers of patent applications as a measure of commercial potential and ultimate success of research. Finally, scientists, like most people, crave opportunities to advance at their universities and most are genuinely enthusiastic about their work and its promise. This enthusiasm may lead researchers to overstate the time to realization or scope of the benefits of stem cell research. This is dangerous in that it sets up the research for failure if it does not deliver these benefits or does not deliver them quickly.[75]

Researchers, then, are stuck between potentially conflicting priorities. They need to bang the drum for their work to get funding and take their experiments further. But if they bang that drum too loud, they risk damaging the credibility of the very science they serve.

All research scientists must 'sell' the value of their work to governments and funding agencies to get the money they need to carry their experiments forward. Stem cell researchers face an even bigger challenge, given the ethical debate that swirls around their science. They are often put in a position of explaining to politicians and funding bodies why investing in stem cell research is worth the risk of incurring the wrath of those who would prefer to see it shut down. As anyone would expect, they employ all of the hypotheticals, the promises of what stem cells might be able to do if their work is properly funded. They produce laundry lists of the diseases that they – quite legitimately – hope to treat or cure some day.

Hard Realities

It is no surprise, then, that the general public gets confused. People absorb media reports about all the things that stem cells can potentially do, but when they go to the doctor they are told that there is nothing for them. People tire of promises. They want results. And many are prepared to look elsewhere when they feel that mainstream medical science can't help them.

The hard reality is that with the notable exception of therapies for blood and immunological disorders, most real-world stem cell treatments are still some time away. It will take years of intensive, painstaking research conducted in rigorously regulated, closely monitored environments before they are available at a clinic near you.

It can take decades of research and many hundreds of millions of dollars to bring a new drug or treatment to the marketplace. For example, it was 1972 when German researcher Harald zur Hausen started working on the theory that cervical cancer is caused by a virus. It took more than ten years for him to prove that two strains of the human papilloma virus (HPV 16 and HPV 18) are responsible for almost three-quarters of all cases of cervical cancer – the second most common cancer among women.

That discovery led to yet more years of work to develop vaccines to defeat the virus. Only in the past few years – after thousands of women around the world took part in randomized controlled clinical trials – have cervical cancer vaccines made it to the market. The time that elapsed from moving the idea from zur Hausen's lab to a legitimate medical breakthrough that is now saving millions of women's lives? About thirty to thirty-five years, all told, when final analysis of clinical tests is taken into consideration.[76]

Till and McCulloch proved the existence of stem cells five decades ago, and their work underpins the principles behind bone marrow transplantation, the medical miracle that has saved hundreds of thousands of lives and that helped E. Donnall Thomas win the Nobel Prize in 1990. But that miracle was some time coming. Thomas began his work in the 1950s, and the procedure we now take for granted only became common practice in clinics in the 1970s and 1980s.

If stem cell science accomplished nothing else, helping to cure some forms of leukemia would stand as a significant step forward in medical science. But the public has come to expect much more from stem cells. Breakthrough discoveries (many of them Canadian-led) of adult stem cells, such as neural, skin, and retinal pluripotent cells, created considerable interest in cell-based therapies. That interest then soared after 1998, when American biologist James Thomson discovered how to isolate and grow human embryonic stem cells. Suddenly the future seemed wide open and full of unlimited opportunities to fight many different diseases with a brand new weapon.

The possibility of stem cell therapies caught the general public's imagination in a way that few other fields of medical research ever have, says Douglas Sipp of the RIKEN Center for Developmental Biology in Kobe, Japan.

'There was a lot of excitement about the future of gene therapy fifteen years ago, but I'm not aware of any case in which a clinic that was claiming to be doing gene therapy opened in a place like Mexico and had flocks of people going there for miracle cures,' says Sipp, who has co-authored academic papers on stem cell tourism and who writes a blog on the subject called *Stem Cell Treatment Monitor.*

'Despite the media excitement and scientific excitement around gene therapy, it didn't attract people. Stem cells, for whatever reason, do. People apparently feel it's something they can understand. There seems to be something about the idea of using cells, rather than chemicals or molecules or gene therapy, that is attractive to people. There's more of a sense that it's commonsensical, that the cells have this benign, almost magical ability to fix what's wrong with whatever person they're put into.'

In 2010, Sipp provided expert commentary to a *60 Minutes* investigation into fraudulent stem cell therapies. He told the television program there are more than two hundred such operations around the world, ranging from those offering 'some version of stem cells for some type of medical condition for which there is no good evidence that stem cells would be safe or effective' to 'thieves preying on the sick and their families.' He feels that many factors have contributed to creating a situation in which unethical and unscrupulous entrepreneurs can exploit the hopes of desperate patients.

'You could put blame on the reporters. You could put blame on the patients for being gullible. You could put blame on the scientists for being overenthusiastic. But at the end of the day none of those things are criminal or harmful to others. But then there are people who are behaving unethically and using that for their own enrichment.'

The controversy surrounding the use of embryonic stem cells has only raised expectations about what stem cells might be able to do, says Sipp. 'It brought out the most extreme opinions on both sides of the argument: that the research was murder or that it was the future source for miracle cures for all kinds of diseases. It did get amplified because of political and legal issues surrounding the research.'

Most governments have regulations in place on the medical uses of stems cells – both adult and embryonic ones. In the United States, for example, the Food and Drug Administration has a comprehensive set of regulations on the use of stem cell–derived or stem cell–based medical products. Not surprisingly, then, countries with less strict rules or with laissez-faire enforcement of existing laws about stem cells have become havens for those who want to do their work without oversight and without undergoing the rigours of randomized controlled clinical trials before offering treatment.

Unfortunately, there is no shortage of people who will not – or feel they cannot – wait for medical researchers to do proper due diligence on stem cell therapies before putting them into the clinic.

Sipp balks at labelling such people stem cell tourists. 'I don't think they are going to [these countries] because they are interested in visiting temples. They are going there because they are compelled by their condition to seek treatment wherever it might be available in the world.' Regardless how they are labelled, such people usually feel that mainstream medical research has failed them. Or even, Sipp suggests, that it is conspiring to prevent them from getting the treatment they need.

'Certainly there are people who feel the regulatory system is inherently too slow,' says Sipp. 'And there are other people who think, more extremely, that there is a kind of conspiracy: that the drug companies are afraid of stem cells because they would hurt their business by curing diseases which right now are being treated by lifelong medication. There are all kinds of wild conspiracy theories. A lot of them include that the regulatory body in whatever country, usually the Food and Drug Administration in the United States, is simply the tool of whatever forces are trying to keep miracle cures from the people. That kind of thinking also sometimes drives people to travel overseas.'

More typical, says Sipp, is the less extreme case: a person with a disease or condition has heard a lot of buzz about stem cells in the media and finds a website for a clinic claiming that it has an effective treatment.

'I generally tell them it's not worth going. Depending on the place, I'll tell them the details of what I know about the company. I track a lot of companies and the individuals associated with them. I'll just give them the information. If I know what [the company's] profit model is, if they are a company that's made tens or hundreds of millions of dollars doing this, I'll say, "Think for yourself. Is this a miracle cure or is it just another guy who's trying to make money off of sick people?"'

For those who might be swayed by others who claim that their condition has been cured or improved by blasts of stem cells at some offshore clinic, Sipp again urges caution. 'It's been shown in experiments that people experience a stronger placebo effect if the treatment costs more money. If you're dealing with something that costs tens of thousands of dollars, which many of these stem cell treatments cost, patients are predisposed to believe that it's going to be effective. Also, many people can't afford it, so they either borrow the money from family or friends or they have community fundraisers or they get money from their church organization. I think that also tends to, if not inflate the reports of positive outcomes, suppress the reports of negative or neutral outcomes. People may be hesitant to come back and tell people they borrowed money from that the whole thing was a scam and that it cost $25,000 to find out.'

For those who would despair, it's important to remember that research is proceeding, however slowly and carefully. There are thousands of clinical trials going on around the world to test the safety and effectiveness of using adult stem cells in treating everything from Alzheimer's disease to damaged hearts to broken knees. Most of the trials involve re-engineering the patient's own stem cells to affect repair. Research into the use of embryonic stem cells is not nearly as far along – not surprising, considering that the first cells were derived only in 1998.

At the time this book was being written, there were only three clinical trials in the works using human embryonic stem cells to treat disease. According to the U.S. National Institutes of Health, the California-based biotechnology company Geron Corporation had begun enrolling patients in a trial to test the safety of using human embryonic stem cells to restore spinal cord function. Another biotech company, also in California, had received permission to begin enrolling patients in two clinical trials. Advanced Cell Technology is in the early stages of investigating the use of retinal cells derived from human embryonic stem cells to treat patients with an eye disease called Statgardt's Macular Dystrophy and those with macular degeneration.[77] In comparison to those three trials, there are more than three thousand clinical trials involving other forms of stem cells, according to the National Institutes of Health.[78]

Stem cell treatments hold great promise for the future. That future can't arrive fast enough for someone who is suffering from a chronic, degenerative, or terminal disease. In the meantime, the age-old caveat will continue to apply: let the buyer beware.

7
The Evil Twin: The Cancer Stem Cell

It is no coincidence that two cancer researchers proved the existence of stem cells. Nor is it a coincidence that it happened in laboratories on the top two floors of a cancer hospital. Cancer research and stem cell research have always walked hand in hand. When they found those bumps on the spleens of the irradiated mice, Jim Till and Ernest McCulloch were part of a team looking for ways to launch a counterattack on leukemia. So, as touched upon earlier in this book, it is not surprising that it is now widely believed – though still disputed by many – that cancer is what happens when good stem cells go bad and become cancer stem cells.

In simple terms, stem cells are the basic building units of the human body. They have the capacity to renew themselves and create progenitor cells, which in turn create the millions of specialized cells that make up a tissue. According to the cancer stem cell hypothesis, the stem cell has, essentially, an evil twin, the cancer stem cell, which also has the ability to renew itself and create progenitor cells, which in turn create the millions of cells that make up a tumour.

The hypothesis is built on the principle that all cancer cells are not created equal. Some are more important than others. At the top of the hierarchy are the cancer stem cells. They start out like normal adult stem cells whose job it is to replace weary or dead cells in a particular organ or tissue (unlike totipotent embryonic stem cells, which have the capacity to create cells for any part of the body). These cancer stem cells are very rare – potentially a one-in-a-million cell depending on the type of cancer. They have the capacity to create new versions of themselves (self-renew) and spawn progenitor cells that, in turn, differentiate into millions of tumour cells.

With normal stem cells, self-renewal, progeneration, and differentiation are all part of how the body regulates itself to keep everything in balance – a state called homeostasis. However, with the cancer stem cell, the whole process is dysfunctional. The differentiated cells are created too abundantly and, according to John Hassell, one of Canada's leading researchers in the field of cancer stem cells, are 'caricatures' of the normal cells required by the organ or tissue where they develop.

'The cancer stem cells spawn these other cells, progenitor-like cells, which have a high proliferative capacity,' says Hassell, the Director of the Centre for Functional Genomics at McMaster University in Hamilton. 'Just as they would if they had descended from a normal stem cell, they go through a differentiation program and attempt to establish as normal cells of the tissue. But because they can't figure it out, the cells sort of look normal but they're not really normal; the tissue's disorganized. It can be a lump or a tumour.'

That cancer appears to parallel processes of normal stem cells seems perfectly logical – and almost obvious. Yet the discovery of cancer stem cells is fairly recent. John Dick, a second-generation Till and McCulloch research descendant via his work with Alan Bernstein and Bob Phillips, accomplished it only in 1994, publishing his findings in a paper in *Nature*.[79]

While Dick's discovery was revolutionary in pinpointing the origin of tumours, it took some time to have an impact. Hassell says that scientists who were working in other areas of cancer research at the time probably assumed that the discovery applied only to the cancer he was investigating: leukemia.

'I think many people thought that what was true for leukemia probably wasn't true for solid tumours and never followed it up,' says Hassell. 'It took over ten years before anyone showed that this was true for anything other than leukemia. The next example was [Stanford University's] Michael Clarke's data in breast cancer – then [Canadians] Peter Dirks and Sheila Singh made their discoveries in brain tumours. It took a hell of a long time for people to pick up on this and show that what was true for hematopoietic-like cancers, leukemias, was also true for solid tumours.'

Indeed, Dirks, who is a neurosurgeon at Toronto's Hospital for Sick Children as well as a stem cell researcher, sought Dick's guidance before embarking on his own research into brain tumours. 'John Dick was at Sick Kids' at that time so, looking for some mentorship ... I arranged a meeting with John and he suggested considering a couple of his papers he had published in *Nature* and *Nature Medicine* identifying the leukemic stem cell in the acute myeloid leukemia.'

The idea wasn't altogether new, Dirks says. 'If you look more carefully at the older literature, which I then started to do, there are important papers published in the early 1980s, really laying some of the groundwork or thought processes of considering cancer stem cells and solid tumours.'

Dirks says that breakthroughs like his were made possible by advances in 'neuro stem cell biology and some tools to culture neuro stem cells, coupled with the emergence of flow cytometry,' which allows researchers to measure and map the size and characteristics of individual cells. 'We had a paper in *Cancer Research* in 2003 and then one in *Nature* in 2004, which showed that we could identify the cell that has these clonogenic properties *in vitro* and then more importantly tumorigenic properties *in vivo*.

'We published our *Nature* paper the year after the paper from Mike Clarke's group showed that you can isolate a tumour-initiating cell from human breast cancer. Our paper was the second such demonstration of prospective sorting for this cell in another solid human cancer, suggesting that the principles laid out years before and more definitively shown by John Dick in leukemia were also applying to solid cancers.'

Like Hassell, Dirks feels that most researchers at the time felt that the cancer stem cell theory applied only to leukemia. 'A lot of people just weren't thinking of considering solid cancers and dissociating them into individual cells and testing the function of those individual cells in a stem cell assay.'

Dick identified cancer stem cells by transplanting human leukemia cells into immune-deficient mice, a process called xenotransplantation. By dividing up the transplanted tumour cells into subsets based on how they expressed proteins, he was able to demonstrate that only one kind – a one-in-a-million cell – was capable of generating tumour production.

Unfortunately, cancer stem cells are exceedingly rare and are also remarkably resistant to what currently constitutes cancer treatment. While their progenitor and differentiated offspring succumb to drugs and radiation, some cancer stem cells may still be standing after they've been hit with the heaviest artillery available in the oncologists' drug arsenal. In technical terms, these cells possess what is called 'a heightened capacity to efflux anticancer drugs.' In other words, these evil twin cells, when exposed to a current anti-cancer drug, can spit some of it right back out.

They are also very good at shrugging off radiation. Hassell says there is a considerable body of scientific literature indicating that cancer stem cells can repair DNA damaged by radiation and carry on. 'The cancer stem cells have a sort of a souped-up DNA repair process or mechanism and any damage that's caused by the radiation is quickly repaired and the cell survives.'

Current therapies are decimating the foot soldiers and squadron leaders of cancer but leaving some of the generals unscathed and fully capable of rebuilding their armies. Armed with this knowledge, many researchers are suggesting that medical science needs to do nothing less than relaunch the war on cancer with cancer stem cells as the key target.

'We may be using therapies that simply don't target these cells,' says Hassell. 'So while you may achieve a transient cure for the patient, it will only be durable if you can knock out the cancer stem cells.'

The call to arms in relaunching the war on cancer has been taken up by two major North American research organizations. In Canada, the Cancer Stem Cell Consortium is bringing together researchers, funding agencies, non-governmental organizations, and private sector partners to coordinate and accelerate cancer stem cell research. At the time this book was being written, the consortium's president was Jim Till. In the United States, the key player is the California Institute for Regenerative Medicine, a state agency established after voters passed Proposition 71 in 2004 and provided it with $3 billion in funding.

The two organizations have pledged to work together, and in 2008, the Canadian government committed $100 million to partnership ventures between Canadian and Californian scientists.

However, while a whole new battlefront has been established in the war on cancer, there is a significant scientific contingent that disputes the cancer stem cell hypothesis. To them, researchers like Dick and Dirks may have miscalculated.

In 2008, Canadian-born stem cell researcher Sean Morrison of the University of Michigan co-authored a paper in *Nature* in which he argued that cancer stem cells are not one in million, but more like one in four. Morrison, who was working with melanoma tumours, suggested that if you alter the xenotransplantation process and use a different type of immunodeficient mouse, you get a different result:

> In limiting dilution assays, approximately 25% of unselected melanoma cells from 12 different patients, including cells from primary and meta-

> static melanomas obtained directly from patients, formed tumours under these more permissive conditions. In single-cell transplants, an average of 27% of unselected melanoma cells from four different patients formed tumours. Modifications to xenotransplantation assays can therefore dramatically increase the detectable frequency of tumourigenic cells, demonstrating that they are common in some human cancers.[80]

Morrison then went further in a 2009 article published online at the Howard Hughes Medical Institute, in which he said that though leukemia may be a special case, in other cancers there are lots of other cells – not just cancer stem cells – that are responsible for making tumours:

> Data from our lab and others indicate that acute and chronic myeloid leukemias appear to follow a cancer stem cell model. In both cases, leukemogenic cells are rare, phenotypically distinct from the vast majority of other leukemia cells, and robustly hierarchically organized. However, it is not clear how generalizable the cancer stem cell model is. In other human and mouse cancers we have studied, including melanoma, tumourigenic capacity is a common attribute of many cancer cells and we have been unable to find any clear evidence of hierarchical organization. Our impression is that the growth and progression of many cancers are driven by many cells rather than by cancer stem cells.[81]

Dick, who welcomes the controversy because he believes it will help stem cell science and cancer research move forward, is unfazed. 'When it's one in four, you can argue that [the tumour cells] are all equal and therefore there's no hierarchy. And if there's no hierarchy, then it's sort of meaningless to talk about a stem cell – every cell is equal. A stem cell only makes sense in the context of hierarchy.'

He argues that what's needed is a finer understanding of cancer stem cells. 'People often think that cancer stem cells are themselves homogeneous. But a lot of work that we've done is indicating that cancer stem cells themselves have variations in their self-renewal capacity. So they all meet the minimal definition but some are able to sustain self-renewal to a higher extent than others.

'A tumour, when it's diagnosed, could be different than a tumour that has relapsed five years later after chemotherapy and surgery. You could have a tumour [with] one cell in a million early on in the evolution of that tumour, whereas when it becomes metastatic it could be a much higher frequency. That's one of the arguments that is being used in the melanoma case of Morrison because he typically used only metastatic disease or high-grade melanoma ... A tumour which can look very, very cancer stem cell–like where you have only a very rare cell, the shape of that hierarchy can change over time, and you can end up with tumours ... where the cells become more and more stem cell–like and the ratio between cancer stem cell to a non-cancer stem cell can change dramatically.'

Dirks says the cancer stem cell hypothesis underpins research in the field of brain cancer. 'There's no group that's ignoring this. There is no group that's not applying stem cell methodologies and stem cell thinking to the study of brain cancer. I think the evidence in brain cancer is fairly strong ... It may not necessarily be a one in a million like John [Dick] has shown in leukemia but still, in general, it's a minority population.'

While the debate carries on, there is great hope for the future of cancer treatment – and new hope for potential cures. Hassell, for one, believes that what's needed now is a major effort to find ways to shut cancer stem cells down. 'Most of my research is focused on trying to find compounds that ultimately can be developed into drugs that kill cancer stem cells. And we've made a lot of progress.'

Scientists such as Hassell want to test different compounds against cancer stem cells to see which ones can slay the cells – without damaging cells around them or having other adverse affects. Testing is being done using high-throughput screening – a process that pools the resources of advanced robotics, sophisticated software, and comprehensive data processing. Essentially, it involves sorting through the compounds to come up with suitable ones to send in to fight cancer stem cells – ones the cells can't spit back out.

'We have shown, and some other investigators have shown, that you can find compounds that kill cancer stem cells,' says Hassell. 'The compound we found was one of among 35,000 in a high-throughput screen to try to identify compounds that would kill cancer stem cells but not normal stem cells. Because all our anti-cancer drugs now kill everything that proliferates. That's why your hair falls out, your intestines go to hell, and your blood supply is low. We're looking for a compound with that specificity or selectivity.'

The process is very slow-going. Hassell says there are millions of compounds to sort through to find those that can kill cancer stem cells but leave other cells unscathed. However, the tedious and time-consuming testing of compounds could hold the key to curing cancer.

8

The Beneficiary

If stem cell science is still a work in progress, there have been some notable successes beyond bone marrow transplantation and advances in cancer treatment. There have been reported cases of immunological disorders such as HIV and Crohn's disease responding well to stem cell treatment. And since 2001, two Ottawa doctors, one of whom is directly linked to the Till and McCulloch scientific lineage, have been pioneering a stem cell treatment for multiple sclerosis. By the close of 2010, two dozen patients had gone through the treatment. Jennifer Molson was one of them.

Looking back, Molson thinks that her disease was always there, lurking in the shadows. All teenagers need plenty of rest, but she could sleep for four days straight, never wanting to get out of bed. Tired all the time, she needed naps to get through a day. When she caught colds, they lingered for weeks or escalated into influenza. She remembers feeling occasional numbness and putting it down to a pinched nerve in her neck or having slept in an awkward position.

In the spring of 1996, the year she turned twenty-one, Molson's left arm went numb and stayed that way. Her hand ignored what her brain was telling it to do. She couldn't retrieve change from her pocket to pay for coffee. She couldn't hold the cup. When an early diagnosis of carpal tunnel syndrome didn't seem to fit the severity of symptoms, she was referred to a neurologist.

Molson was working full time and going to school at night, training to be a police officer. She had started dating Aaron, someone she knew from high school, and it looked like it could be a serious relationship. Her whole life was spread out before her. She was admitted to hospital and scheduled for an MRI.

'They told me I had multiple sclerosis. It was one of those, "My whole life flashed before my eyes" kind of things. When I came back in the room after the diagnosis, Aaron was there and I told him. Then I said, "There's the door." What did I know about MS? Just what I remembered from school, from doing MS Readathons for wheelchairs. No one in my family or anyone I knew had ever had MS. I thought the worst. I thought, "My God, a wheelchair."'

It turned out that her worst fears were justified.

Multiple sclerosis is an autoimmune disease – a disorder in which the body's immune system, which is supposed to defend against infection and outside invaders, turns against its own healthy tissue. With MS, the immune system goes after myelin, the sheath that surrounds the cells in the central nervous system (the brain and the spinal cord), causing inflammation and damage. The effect is such that the nerve cells can't communicate so that messages from the brain – to move a hand or shift a leg – can't get through.

The list of potential symptoms of MS is a daunting one, ranging from 'brain fog' and loss of balance to difficulty in walking and optic nerve inflammation. Jennifer displayed a fairly common symptom before she was diagnosed: useless hand syndrome.

According to the MS Society of Canada, there are four kinds of MS, varying in severity of symptoms and frequency of 'episodes' or 'attacks.' A common form is relapsing/remitting MS, in which the disease waxes and wanes. Episodes can take hold over a few hours or a few days. They can stay a weekend or may stick around for a season. When an episode subsides, symptoms can disappear and life may return to pre-attack normal. Remission can last a few months, even a few years.

With primary progressive MS the symptoms gradually get worse with no oases of remissions. There may be some stabilization, but this kind of MS is marked by slow decline and increasing disability.

Secondary progressive MS seems to bloom like an noxious weed out of relapsing/remitting MS. The time between episodes evaporates as symptoms become unrelenting. Sporadic flare-ups and slight improvements may still occur, but this form of MS is marked by more and more disability, less and less mobility.

There is also progressive relapsing MS, a more rare form that generally means a steep and steady decline into disability.

Molson says she originally had relapsing/remitting MS and, for a while, she showed classic symptoms of this form of the disease: her useless hand syndrome that came on in May disappeared in August, when full use of her left arm returned. For a time, anyway. Her episodes came and went.

It did not take long, however, for things to get worse. She quit the police training program soon after her diagnosis but continued to work full time. Then she cut back to part-time work. She quit driving because she couldn't grip the steering wheel or feel it in her hands. She lost the ability to write with her right hand and tried using her left. She was weak and exhausted much of the time and walking became increasingly difficult. Eventually, she quit work altogether.

'By February of 2001, I was not well. My brain stem was affected and I had vertigo all the time. By September, I started my rapid decline, and by November, I was living at the Rehab Centre at the General Campus of the Ottawa Hospital, learning how to live with my disability.' Her boyfriend Aaron – who did not walk out the door – had to cut her food and feed her, help her in and out of the shower, and dry her hair. She was incapable of putting socks on her own feet.

'I was twenty-six,' says Molson. 'I could go home on weekends, but somebody had to be with me all the time. I was using two forearm crutches or a walker. Within five years I had gone from working full time and going to school to living in a rehab centre with twenty-four-hour care. That was one of my rock bottoms.'

At that point, Molson had not met Dr Harry Atkins, a bone marrow transplant specialist who, along with treating leukemia patients at the Ottawa Hospital, is a world-renowned medical researcher. A quiet man who speaks precisely and eschews exaggeration, he conducts research because he finds it 'frustrating to be limited by the tools we have in medicine right now.' There are, he says, just too many unanswered questions.

During the early 1990s, Atkins had trained with Norman Iscove, a former McCulloch PhD student, and worked with Hans Messner, the bone marrow transplant wunderkind whom McCulloch had personally recruited to the Ontario Cancer Institute from Germany. Atkins became intrigued by the possibility, championed by Italian researcher Alberto Marmont, of using bone marrow transplantation to treat autoimmune diseases. 'People were transplanting patients with leukemia and some of them also had autoimmune diseases,' he remembers. 'These autoimmune diseases would get better along with the leukemia.'

Atkins met with Marmont and other like-minded researchers and clinicians, then came back to Ottawa and started investigating bone marrow transplantation for diseases such as rheumatoid arthritis. 'It's lost in the depths of my memory, but somehow I had a conversation with a neurologist who said, "MS is really an autoimmune disease, maybe you should do this for MS." That's really how it came about. Around 1997, we started thinking we should do something along those lines. It took a long time to do due diligence, to bring a group together, to get a protocol written, to get grant funding. It has been a slow process all the way along. Probably that's for the better because that way it's as safe as possible for the patients.'

Atkins works with Mark Freedman, Jennifer's neurologist since October 1996. As was the case with Till and McCulloch, it is an unusual partnership of two men from different fields. 'Typically, transplant physicians and neurologists look after very different patient populations,' says Atkins. Together, they devised the clinical trial to treat patients with the most severe forms of MS – people such as Jennifer Molson, for whom life in a wheelchair is a virtual certainty.

'MS is an autoimmune disease where the immune system is attacking a patient's brain,' says Atkins. 'The simple concept behind our treatment is, "Let's just get rid of the old immune system and put back the seeds, let a new one grow and hope that it won't learn the same lesson." Because stem cells don't carry over immunologic memory. That's really what we have tried to do. We had a track record for doing transplants for leukemia and knew how we could damage the immune system to remove it. We just applied the lessons we learned in care of patients with leukemia and applied them to this new setting.'

While the concept is quite simple, the execution is anything but. The therapy that Atkins and Freedman have devised has pushed the limits of medical technology. 'We're giving high-dose chemotherapy; we're purifying stem cells. These are cutting-edge techniques and we've put them together. It needs a lot of attention and care to make sure our patients come through this safely.' Indeed, as treatments go, it is at the extreme end of aggressive and, as Atkins describes it, 'was quite different in scale than anything the neurology community was doing for MS at the time.'

According to Freedman, the goal was to eliminate every single potential MS-causing cell from the patient's body. The protocol they came up with was patterned on the complete bone marrow ablation performed on patients who receive mismatched bone marrow – patients for whom failure to kill all the pre-existing marrow cells could prove fatal. 'We also wanted to be able to deal with the cells that had already gained entry to the central nervous system, because if we didn't it was only a matter of time before those cells worked their way back out and restimulated the disease.'

Atkins and Freedman devised a treatment in which the patient's immune system is completely laid to waste by chemotherapy and removed. Then it is reseeded with the patient's own purified and fortified stem cells, which are extracted earlier in the process.

'We have a machine called a stem cell selector,' says Atkins. 'We use a monoclonal antibody [an immune protein produced from a single clone of cells] with little iron filings on it that recognizes the stem cells. We mix the stem cells with the antibodies and pass them through a magnetic field so that the stem cells are all held up. We wash away all the immune cells and all the other cells we don't want. Then we release the magnetic field and the stem cells are collected in a separate container.'

Disease Running Amok

Molson first heard about the stem cell transplant trial from Freedman in February 2001 while at the Ottawa Hospital's MS clinic for steroid treatments. 'It was February and at that point the study was still in the recruiting process, just getting up and running. I guess I'd read in the paper before about bone marrow transplants. I remember thinking there was no way I'd ever do that. Like, you've got to be crazy. But me, in 2001, I was there. I wasn't feeling any relief between my episodes. Obviously, I was going down. And between February and November, it got much worse.'

Freedman recalls the February conversation when Molson was having her steroid treatment and being attended to by one of his team. 'I pulled my fellow aside and said, "You know, this is buying her a little bit of time, but we're going to need to do something more definitive for her or she's going to be very disabled, very quickly." She showed all the signs that her disease was running amok.'

He suggests that trying to delineate between Molson's early-stage MS and the later extreme version that qualified her for the trial is an exercise in futility. 'Jennifer and the other patients in this trial are very unique and for me to say they're relapsing/remitting or secondary progressive – I think the point is moot. They all had a very aggressive form of MS, meaning that almost every time they had another relapse they were left with residual deficits. And once you start to see that, you're dealing with someone who is essentially running out of their reserves.'

In deciding whether Molson qualified for the trial, Freedman says it was a matter of realizing she was in serious trouble and not responding to the usual regimen of drugs that MS patients receive for relief. The question he asked himself was, 'Have I given her a fair opportunity to respond to the traditional drugs? We hadn't really treated her all that long before she started to have problems, even on the traditional drugs.'

In May of 2002, Molson began the new, experimental treatment with a brief stay in hospital. 'They took a litre of my bone marrow, harvested from my pelvis bone. That was my back-up bone marrow – in case my stem cells didn't work, they would just give me my old stuff back.'

She was back in the hospital in June. She remembers being 'hooked up to the stem cell collection machine for several hours' as part of the treatment. It involved taking blood from a site on her arm, running it through a machine, and rerouting it back to her through her chest. 'They cycled my total body blood mass thirty-two times.' The process yielded a small bag of stem cells that, once purified and fortified, would be put to work rebuilding her immune system. She was not impressed by the look of them. 'They were grey, ugly looking things, very cloudy. Not very nice.'

There were ten days of intense chemo. 'There was an oral chemo, one hundred twenty-nine pills a day for four days. I don't have a very strong stomach, so they'd wake me up to eat some crackers and take the pills. When that was done, I had four days of cyclophosphamide [an intravenous chemo known for causing hair loss and nausea]. And they put me on this stuff called ATG [anti-thymocyte globulin]. That's the chemo that Dr Atkins said, "This can cause all your organs to shut down."'

Because the treatment annihilates the immune system, it pulls a patient very close to death. In fact, the participant who followed Molson in the study did not survive the chemotherapy stage. 'We knew the risks were there,' says Molson. 'I knew the possibility [of death] was there. But my disease was so bad.'

Boyfriend Aaron had a hard time of it. 'After three days, with me just having the chemo, he was thinking, "Oh my God, she's not going to make it." He said I looked really bad.' Aaron agrees: 'There were a couple of days where she was just grey, like pavement. I didn't think she was going to live through some of the nights. The treatment was that intense.'

Molson's stem cell transplant took place on 4 July 2002, a date she now celebrates as her second birthday. After so much preparation and hardship, it was anticlimactic. It only took about twenty minutes for the liquid stem cells to travel through the intravenous drip and into her veins. It smelled so much like sour milk that Aaron had to leave the room to avoid being sick.

Then Molson hit another rock bottom. 'I had one of those tubes that goes through your nose and down your throat. I got really nauseous and I went to the bathroom to be sick. I got my head in the garbage can and actually threw up the tube. I had to pull the emergency cord because I didn't know what to do. And twenty nurses came running into the room. I remember thinking, "Oh my God, what am I doing?"

'That was probably a week after the chemo. That was around day fifteen and I was in hospital, probably twenty-one to twenty-five days. I went in in June and I wasn't out until around July 15. I went in weighing one hundred and thirty pounds. I dropped to one hundred and ten. I'm a little over five feet, nine inches tall. My Mom said I looked like I'd come out of a concentration camp. I was all sunken in and grey.'

Molson did not immediately respond to the transplant treatment. 'My whole bone marrow system was gone. I had to have blood transfusions and platelets. My white cell count was zero. It took several days before it went back up to zero-point-five. A week and a half later it was three.'

It was a harrowing experience. Bald from the chemo, physically wrecked, underweight and weak, she developed a blood infection in the hospital. She remembers being profoundly depressed. She convinced the medical staff to let her go home, even though she was still on 'this super-antibiotic that will kill anything. They let me do it. But I still had to come back every day to check my blood levels.'

Eventually, Molson began to get better. As recoveries go, however, it wasn't the stuff of Hollywood movies. She did not wake up one morning, throw back the covers, and walk into her garden to gather bouquets of roses. It was a long, slow, series of improvements and setbacks. It was difficult: 'I threw up for a year after.'

Initially, Molson had to return to the hospital every day, then once a month for her immune booster. 'So here I am, bald. And everybody thinks I have cancer, because I'm on the cancer floor. And they ask "What sort of cancer do you have?" And I don't have cancer. And I'm thinking, "Why did I do this to myself? I was fine." These people have to do this to live. It took me a really long time to wrap my head around the fact that I was doing this to live too.'

She developed shingles – a viral disease marked by a painful skin rash with blisters – like a highly localized chicken pox. Hers was on her face, and it sent her back to hospital for antiviral treatment. But even feeling better had its hardships. 'You go through cycles. Highs and then depressions. MS is your whole life, knowing you're going down. Then you're going up and you don't know how to cope with being better.'

Molson remembers her life coming back to her little by little. 'I would be doing stuff and then I'd say, "Wait a second. I'm actually carrying books down stairs without holding on to the railing." Or I'd realize, "I didn't have a nap today. I've been awake since seven." "I'm standing in the kitchen and I don't need to sit down while I'm making dinner." It was gradual. I was living in a condo then, so my mailbox was in the building. I went to get the mail and I realized I left my canes in the apartment. That's when I knew that I was getting better.'

On 21 June 2003, eleven months after her treatment, Jennifer married Aaron. She went the whole day without using her canes. She danced at the reception.

Freedman says that the goal of the Freedman/Atkins study was to prevent patients from further deterioration from the progressive nature of their MS; it was not to diminish patients' disabilities. 'The getting-better part was totally unanticipated. We thought we could control it. I felt we might be able to control it for a while, but I thought the most interesting part of this experiment would be that if we effectively re-booted the entire immune and white blood cell system, and if we were vigilant enough, we might see the first signs of MS as it unfolds and get a clue to what causes the disease. So, fully expecting patients to redevelop their disease, our protocol was to be monitoring them every month and doing immunological studies and MRIs and exams to try to pick up the first signs of disease.

'We failed. Nobody redeveloped the disease. So Plan B became: How long is this going to last? We went on for two years, three years, four years. I went to my colleagues and asked, "What will convince you that we've wiped out the disease? How long do we have to wait?" They said that most chemo will buy people up to five years, so if you can do a median survival of five years, we'll believe you. We hit the median survival of five years this year, so we're putting the publication together.'

Not all of the twenty-four participants in the trial got better. But, importantly, most did not get any worse. None had further active inflammation from the MS. Jennifer Molson was not the first patient to show signs of improvement, but her return to good health has been the most dramatic.

'I had no idea that she had been getting better,' says Freedman, 'but when she came in for an appointment wearing heels, I went, "Stop, what is happening here? She's recovering function." This was two years from the transplant, so no one could say that it was the transplant regimen or the chemotherapy that was responsible. Something has kick-started this repair, and I don't know what that is.

'We have reapplied for funding, not so much to extend the trial but to understand why some people are actually getting better. We started seeing things I'd never seen improve. Once people have lost their balance and they're uncoordinated and they require walkers, I don't expect to see them ever walk independently again. But that's what started to happen. I wouldn't expect someone who's been blind from optic neuritis for three or four years to suddenly start seeing out of that eye again, and that's what happened.

'Is it the fact that we have just completely stopped a person's disease and as a result that has allowed them to repair? That's possible. Is it the fact that we put in stem cells that we thought were only going to repopulate their bone marrow and redo their hematopoietic and immunological systems, but they're actually capable of doing more? We now know that bone marrow–derived stem cells can become any cell in the body. Have they become brain cells? Have they actually helped to repair or stimulate the cells in the brain to get the job done? Or are they themselves turning into brain cells capable of repair? Those are the things that we've been trying to work out.'

Atkins says that further study is required. 'We are talking with other people throughout the world who are working on this problem about doing a more robust trial, a randomized controlled trial to develop stronger evidence that this is an effective treatment. We're in the preliminaries of that.'

He still does not use the term cure. 'We don't know that. Time will tell. It's too soon to be able to tell us that. It certainly is not a treatment for everybody. There are risks involved. For the right patient with the right kind of MS, we think this is beneficial. But we're still accumulating evidence and will be for a long time. There might be easier ways of treating patients with less severe MS, ways that are less risky. But knowing what we know now, it has implications for how to approach MS. We're looking to change the natural course of that disease.'

Molson has resumed a full and active life. She now feels better than ever. She went back to work, first part time, then full time, and now sometimes puts in twelve-hour days in her job at the hospital, where she looks after scheduling for cancer patients.

'I downhill ski. I drive a standard – hey, I can shift. Isn't that crazy? I can skate, but not very well. I'm more hesitant now. Falling hurts more now. I never used to have feeling, so it never really bothered me to fall. I can dance but not well. I'm like Julia Louis-Dreyfus on *Seinfeld:* I have no rhythm. That was always the case. I'm not on any medication. Just hormone therapy because I'm in menopause from the chemo. Other than that, I'm on nothing.'

Molson lived with MS for six years. At the time this book was written, she had been clear of the disease for more than eight years. 'Am I cured? I like to use that word. They don't like to use that word. They're calling it a lasting remission. I'm very lucky. I count my blessings every day. I've got a second chance at life. How many people get that?'

In medical research, dividends are often paid out long after the initial investment. In this case, the payoff came more than four decades after the fact. The results that Atkins and Freedman are getting are directly traceable to the Till and McCulloch discoveries. Iscove and Messner learned from Till and McCulloch. Atkins learned from Iscove and Messner, took the knowledge to Ottawa, and shared it with Freedman. And Jennifer Molson, the beneficiary of those discoveries and the knowledge transfer, got her life back.

9

The Future

The revolution in regenerative medicine began not with an explosion, but with a quiet murmur of curiosity expressed by Ernest McCulloch when he observed bumps on the spleens of his irradiated mice. It was a discovery of monumental importance then, for it provided the underpinning principles for bone marrow transplantation and led to leap-ahead advances in the treatment of leukemia and the understanding of cancer. Quite likely, however, its greatest impact is yet to come.

In March 2009, when he signed an executive order to reverse the Bush administration's strict limits on human embryonic stem cell research, U.S. President Barak Obama admitted that 'at this moment, the full potential of stem cell research remains unknown, and it should not be overstated.' But the possibilities are simply too great, Obama said, to leave unexplored. 'Scientists believe these tiny cells may have the potential to help us understand and possibly cure some of our most devastating diseases and conditions. To regenerate a severed spinal cord and lift someone from a wheelchair. To spur insulin production and spare a child from a lifetime of needles. To treat Parkinson's, cancer, heart disease, and others that affect millions of Americans and the people who love them. But that potential will not reveal itself on its own. Medical miracles do not happen simply by accident. They result from painstaking and costly research, from years of lonely trial and error, much of which never bears fruit.'

Given that Till and McCulloch made their pivotal discoveries fifty years ago, the question could fairly be asked: Why are those 'years of lonely trial and error' not a thing of the past? What has borne fruit? Why have scientists not solved more riddles about disease, based on the solutions that Till and McCulloch produced? Do the wheels of medical science turn that slowly?

Yes and no. Till and McCulloch were not out to regenerate nerve tissue damaged by Parkinson's disease when they were charting the proliferation of colony-forming units in a mouse spleen. They were, in fact, focused on coming up with an antidote to radiation sickness and findings ways to treat leukemia. They were not thinking about diabetes or heart disease or spinal cord repair. They were working with blood. And even though they were redefining the principles of one area of human biology, other researchers outside their field did not look at those findings and consider the potential applications. They might not even have known about them.

'The hematologists who were in research recognized the importance,' says Ron Worton, founder of the Stem Cell Network and former Till postdoc. 'A few other people recognized the importance, but people working in liver, or people working on the brain, or people working on other tissues or organs probably didn't even read the papers at the time, so it would have had little impact in that regard.'

Other things had to occur, other discoveries had to be made, before those potential connections could be established, says Worton. 'I think the recognition that [the work] is extremely important in a much, much broader sense didn't come until 1998, when two things happened: embryonic stem cells were discovered in humans, and it became possible to grow human stem cells in cell culture. Then, all of a sudden, people started to say, "Hey, maybe we can use this for therapy," and that's when the rest of the scientific community sat up and took notice. And that, quickly, within two years, meant that everyone in the world, at least in the Western world, was reading about stem cells in the newspaper every other day.'

Viewed that way, stem cell science is not a continuous fifty-year research exercise. There are significant gaps in those five decades. It took other discoveries well beyond the realm of hematology – though many were based on Till and McCulloch's early assays – to kick-start what has come to be known as regenerative medicine. It took the American James Thomson's isolation of human embryonic stem cells in 1998 to awaken the world to the possibilities. It took developments in other areas, particularly the closely related field of genetics, to uncover the possibilities for new therapies. And it took technological advances, especially the application of computer wizardry to the analysis of cells, to open new doors and make what once was impossible now seem quite probable.

The pace at which medical science is moving is subjective: it varies according to where you are standing. 'It depends on how you measure progress, says Gordon Keller, the Director of Toronto's McEwen Centre for Regenerative Medicine. 'In society's eyes ... yes, it is slow. But if you're racing to compete with everybody, it's going very, very fast. The ability to take a cell and turn it into a stem cell and turn those stem cells into heart cells, blood cells, liver cells, and pancreatic cells, it's doable – every day we do it. So in that sense, it's going very fast. But for the patient waiting for new cells for repair, I can understand how that's frustrating and perceived as a very slow, slow process.'

In some ways, however, if the future has not quite arrived, it's definitely coming soon. The debate is about when.

'In three to five years, I would not be surprised if stem or progenitor cell transplantation was already part of the routine treatment of acute myocardial infarction [heart attack],' Duncan Stewart, CEO and Scientific Director of the Ottawa Health Research Institute, explained in e-mail correspondence. 'Ten years from now, I think there is little doubt that regenerative approaches will be part of the mainstay for the treatment for many chronic heart diseases.'

Working at the intersection of cardiology and regenerative medicine, Stewart makes his predictions based on tests and trials that have already shown promising results. 'We are still in the very early stages of translating fairly simple, self-donated adult cell therapy strategies into the clinical arena,' he said, 'concentrating on a select number of targets that may be particularly amenable to this approach. For example, heart attack may be such a target, since it affords an opportunity for cellular therapies to modify injury and improve healing before the heart has become irreversibly scarred and weakened.'

According to Stewart, more than 1,500 patients have already been treated in various cell therapy trials; and systematic reviews of all available clinical data confirm 'highly significant, albeit modest, benefit in terms of improved cardiac function and reduced scarring.' To his way of thinking, 'there is no question that the benefit is clinically important and, if it can be shown to be reproducible in a pivotal trial, could be rapidly adopted as an adjunct procedure in patients who have suffered large heart attacks.'

If the treatment of heart disease is poised to become the next clinical application of stem cell science, diabetes therapies likely will not be far behind. President Obama's projection that stem cells could someday spare a child from a lifetime of needles could be fairly close to becoming a reality.

A devastating disease that afflicts millions of people, diabetes results from insufficient production of the hormone insulin from pancreatic beta cells. Insulin is required to allow the sugar we consume to enter cells of the body as a source of energy.

'For patients with type 1 diabetes, and approximately one-third of those with type 2 diabetes, insulin replacement remains essentially the same as it was when Canadians discovered insulin about ninety years ago – needle and syringe,' wrote Timothy Kieffer of UBC in e-mail correspondence. 'The routine of several insulin injections per day along with multiple checks of blood sugar is cumbersome and inadequate, such that patients with diabetes typically suffer from debilitating complications of the disease and have reduced lifespan.'

In 2000, the Edmonton Protocol established that transplantation of a few teaspoons of insulin-producing cells obtained from donors can effectively treat diabetes. The cells do not even need to be put back into the pancreas. As long as they can be injected somewhere with sufficient blood supply, they can survive, detect increasing blood sugar levels, and release the appropriate amount of insulin. That approach, however, remains limited because the process of isolating insulin-producing cells from the pancreas of organ donors requires highly specialized and costly techniques.

'Stem cells hold considerable promise for making this treatment widely available,' said Kieffer. 'They have virtually unlimited expansion potential and can be converted to any cell type in the body, under the right conditions.' Researchers are already able to make large amounts of insulin-producing cells in the laboratory. 'Preclinical studies are under way to ensure the cells are safe and release the appropriate amount of insulin when exposed to sugar. Undoubtedly further refinements in the process are required, but future prospects of this approach look very promising.'

If Kieffer is optimistic about freeing diabetics from daily injections, Jacques Tremblay, a neuroscientist at Laval University, is just as confident that within a decade people with various hereditary diseases such as muscular dystrophy will be treated with their own genetically corrected stem cells. 'The stem cells used for such treatments will be either tissue-specific – cells derived from a muscle and able to repair the muscles – or non–tissue-specific, such as mesenchymal stem cells [those able to differentiate into a variety of cells].'

Tremblay wrote in an e-mail that he expects that induced pluripotent stem (iPS) cells will be tapped as a key source of non–tissue-specific progenitors because they can be differentiated into all kinds of cells. He sees a day in the not too distant future when the cells derived from a patient with an inherited disease will be genetically corrected and proliferated in cultures and then put back in the organs of the people from whom they originated. 'As they would be autologous cells containing human genes, immunosuppression will not be required.'

In the realm of cancer, Sheila Singh of McMaster University's Stem Cell and Cancer Research Institute thinks that a much better understanding of brain tumour development will soon emerge, built on the foundational work done in leukemia by pioneers such as John Dick.

'Although the cancer stem cell hypothesis has captured the imaginations of scientists, clinicians, patients, and the general public due to its plausibility in explaining the clinical course of the disease, its applications are still developing,' explained Singh in e-mail correspondence. 'The greatest advances toward clinical therapeutics have been made in leukemic stem cells. The study of cancer stem cells in solid tumours lags behind leukemia by several decades, and our understanding of the hierarchy of neural stem cells, and by comparison brain cancer stem cells, is still quite rudimentary.'

She expects scientists' understanding of brain cancer stem cells to begin to advance more quickly as researchers build on the footings put in place by leukemia studies. 'The hope for advancement toward diagnostic and therapeutic targets lies at the crossroads of human genetic studies and stem cell and developmental biology,' she said. Melding the tools these fields have to offer 'will uncover the molecular secrets that lie within the cellular heterogeneity of brain tumours.'

To Allen Eaves, founding Director of the world-famous Terry Fox Lab in Vancouver, the target is obvious. 'The ultimate goal is to cure cancer. That's what it's all about.'

In 1993, Eaves founded STEMCELL Technologies Inc. to provide standardized, high-quality, tissue culture media and cell separation reagents for the Terry Fox Lab as well as for research colleagues around the world. The burgeoning firm employs more than four hundred people and in 2010 generated sales of $50 million. Significant amounts of the revenue, however, are ploughed back into research, largely through the Stem Cell Network, one of Canada's Networks of Centres of Excellence. 'It would probably be somewhere between $5 to $6 million,' he says.

From the point of view of an entrepreneur providing the 'picks and shovels for the stem cell gold rush,' Eaves sees a future that looks very promising. 'Stem cell research, as pioneered so well by Till and McCulloch, is an incredibly hot area,' he says. 'Almost anything you can conceive of biologically is probably possible, not only in cancer research, but also in the new areas of tissue engineering and regenerative medicine.'

Bioengineering the Future

Leo Behie of the University of Calgary would agree that remarkable changes are in the works. In the near future, he wrote in an e-mail, stem cell therapy procedures for a number of serious medical conditions such as Parkinson's disease, Type 1 diabetes, and multiple sclerosis will most likely occur in the surgical suites of hospitals, courtesy of advances in bioreactor technology.

Behie, the founding Director of the Pharmaceutical Production Research Facility, is developing new bioreactor protocols for growing and characterizing human stem cells and progenitor cells for tissues and organs. He works on specific strategies for expanding human neural precursor cells, iPS cells, and mesenchymal stem cells harvested from human tissues, including bone marrow and pancreatic islets.

'I predict that stem/progenitor cells will be produced within a bioreactor room located within the suite itself and then these cells or their differentiated progeny will be transported to the operating room for transplantation. Within the bioreactor room, the final production of the cell will be carried out in computer-controlled bioreactors to ensure the production of high-quality cells in a standardized and reproducible bioprocess.'

There are, however, hurdles to be cleared before stem cell therapies are readily available in hospital surgical suites, wrote Behie, with challenges to be addressed in regard to cell culture media, cell-handling procedures, and bioreactor protocols.

What is becoming increasingly important, says Peter Zandstra of the University of Toronto's Institute of Biomaterials and Biomedical Engineering, is understanding the context of how stem cells function, which requires thinking very small.

'Stem cells live in our bodies in very defined micro-environments,' says Zandstra, who is also a McEwen Centre investigator. 'We're trying to design micro-fabricated devices that mimic the stem cell niche – the micro-environment. We can use biomaterials, polymer chemistry, and micro-fabrication technologies similar to those that are used in the computer chip generation area to design stem cell niches so that we can better control stem cells and learn about the underlying molecular principles that they use to integrate signals and make decisions.'

Understanding the micro-environment in which stem cells operate has potential applications for treating cancer, which occurs when stem cells go dysfunctional, or for manipulating stem cells *in situ* (as they exist the body) for regenerative medicine purposes. 'If we understand what regulates stem cell fate in the niche, then we can perturb that niche to get stem cell growth or stem cell differentiation to control specific responses,' says Zandstra. 'Once we understand the complex language that the micro-environment uses to regulate stem cell fate, we can design new materials or chemical strategies to modulate the niche and control stem cell fate.'

Building a Powerhouse

When Rob and Cheryl McEwen lost two close family members to cancer, they got a close-up look at the state of health care. 'We spent a lot of time in hospitals during those illnesses and we saw first hand what our hospitals are dealing with and the huge demand on the medical system,' says Cheryl. 'There's just not enough space and not enough staff. We wondered how on earth our medical system would be able to handle the baby boomers coming through the doors. How, once that big demographic bulge hits those hospital doors, will we be able to cope?'

Rob, who founded Goldcorp, one of the world's most successful gold mining companies, and Cheryl, a successful businesswoman, decided they wanted to do something that could make a significant and lasting difference in health care. Regenerative medicine and stem cell research caught their attention.

'We had the opportunity and the ability to do something to help, so we explored the areas of greatest need,' says Cheryl. 'We felt that if we could enable Toronto's very strong scientific talent with funding to harness the power of stem cells, we would be able to accelerate collaborative research for many diseases and improve treatments and health care dramatically.'

So far, the couple has donated $21 million to create the McEwen Centre for Regenerative Medicine. It has quickly become a research powerhouse, with many of the top stem cell scientists in Canada and the world on a roster of investigators led by Gordon Keller, whom the McEwens helped recruit from New York. McEwen Centre teams are working on projects that include the development of fully functioning heart tissue for grafting onto damaged hearts, repair of spinal cord injuries using nerve stem cells, restoration of vision lost due to diabetes and macular degeneration, and healing of chronic wounds.

The goal, she says, is to accelerate successes in the lab so that they generate breakthrough treatments in the clinic. 'We call these our Acceleration Awards, and they have time-sensitive reviews and are expected to obtain results within eighteen to twenty-four months.'

The plan is also to commercialize the intellectual property generated from McEwen Centre projects to make further research self-sustaining. 'As a country, Canada has been very successful in publishing intellectual property but not in commercializing it. We hope to change that through our biotech innovations.'

She sees an opportunity to the reduce the enormous costs of developing drugs by using organs and tissues generated from stem cells as testing materials. That could streamline current lengthy and expensive clinical trials. 'Wouldn't it be great to find out in the early stages about a problem with a drug and fix it, or move on to the next drug? That's where we see the benefit in bringing down health care costs and bringing down the cost of drugs.'

McEwen also predicts that the research will lead to the emergence of personalized medicine. 'We will be able to take your own cells, turn them into your heart cells in the lab, and see which heart medication is going to be best for you.'

Beyond bringing down the costs of drugs and personalizing drug therapies, she sees stem cells as becoming the source material for treatments, which could take some pressure off operating rooms and go a long way toward easing the strain on heath care. 'When doctors can deploy your own stem cells, they won't necessarily have to operate on you. There will be ways to receive the stem cell therapy without invasive surgery.'

Man In Motion

While the McEwens envision regenerative medicine as easing the health care burden, Rick Hansen, who wheeled his way around the world in the mid-1980s Man In Motion World Tour, sees stem cell science as holding out the best hope for repairing spinal cord injury.

'There are two big mysteries,' says Hansen, whose foundation has raised more than $245 million to raise awareness and fund research.

'How do we cause the spinal cord to regrow? Great strides are being made in that area. They've proven the spinal cord can regrow. Secondly, once damage has taken place, there are often lost cells and fundamental damage, with cyst cavities that form in the spine, preventing reconnection. The idea of introducing cell replacement capacity offers hope for spinal cord injury, not just for those who are newly injured but also for those who have been injured for many years and who have a cyst cavity. There needs to be a way to stimulate growth across that cavity and replace the lost material. This is where stem cell science has some of the most unbelievable possibilities.'

Hansen realizes that as a field of scientific investigation, regenerative medicine is still in its early days, with no quick fixes in sight. And from his wheelchair perspective, he can understand the frustration over how slowly breakthroughs in repairing spinal injury in mice seem to translate into clinical treatments for human beings. But he looks at second- and third-generation scientists building on Till and McCulloch's pioneering work and sees cures coming in the medium to long term.

'In 2010 we marked our twenty-fifth anniversary of the Man In Motion World Tour. I'd like to think we're halfway down the road toward our ultimate goal of finding a cure for spinal cord injury. Canadians have really pushed the envelope in neural stem cells with Samuel Weiss and Freda Miller on the skin stem cell side. They're moving toward preclinical stages in the lab and within five years we may start to see some really high-end, high-quality clinical trials that are more than just preliminary studies. It could lead into very hopeful phases with patients to determine whether this is working.'

What's crucial is to make sure that scientists around the world are working in collaboration, not in competition. Hansen advocates for a global registry for clinical trials in regenerative medicine, so that advances at one lab can be repeated at other sites.

'We've seen the Chinese also making regenerative medicine a strategic priority. I wouldn't be surprised if one day in the next ten years a Nobel Prize comes out of China in this field, but it's also important that China become part of a global fraternity in this ethical framework. That's one of the innovations we're working on with the Rick Hansen Institute: to create that ethical framework to ensure that multiple centres around the world are collaborating. When great hope is translated into real possibilities, we want that potential to be applied in a global network and registry for clinical trials to get as many centres to participate so that we can validate effectiveness and move to the next level.'

Hansen, who is friends with actor and stem cell campaigner Michael J. Fox, is heartened by what he sees happening in the United States. 'President Obama has done extraordinary work in exercising leadership with opening up stem cell research in the United States. Any time the U.S. gets involved in anything like this it adds more potential and capacity and it positions Canada to be a great partner.'

He knows there is 'some heavy slogging ahead' before researchers reach that next level. 'But there's real hope. We're all betting that neural cell replacement for spinal cord injury is possible. Spinal cord research is so complex. It's never going to come from one silver bullet discovery. It will come from a combination of discoveries and therapies that deal with neural regeneration, reconnection across the injured area, and functional recovery.'

Time and Timing

Sir John Bell, Regius Chair of Medicine at Oxford University, believes that Till and McCulloch's discovery of stem cells is only going to become more significant in the twenty-first century. But he urges patience. 'In terms of application to clinical practice, my belief is it is going to be relevant and probably increasingly relevant. The time frame that I think you have to project to get huge impact in clinical practice is more like twenty years from now rather than ten. We're a long way from using this methodology widely in clinical practice. That's just what happens: everybody always is too enthusiastic about how quickly it's all going to happen. It never happens that fast. But then, when it bites, it really bites.'

But if time is a factor, so is timing. Modern medical science has neutralized many diseases that used to kill millions. Smallpox has been eradicated. Polio has been banished from much of the world. There are global efforts under way to disarm malaria. Measles and rubella can be prevented and controlled. Says Bell: 'Given that many of the causes of acute mortality in young populations are now being controlled globally, and the big burden of disease is very largely degenerative diseases of one sort or another, it seems unlikely that we're not going to have lots of applications in virtually every organ system for regenerative activity.'

To predict the future is to risk ridicule. Fifty years later, the world still laughs about the Decca executive who, when rejecting The Beatles, suggested that guitar music was on the way out. Inventor Lee De Forest, considered to be one of the fathers of the electronic age, did not see much of a future for television. In health research, Pierre Pachet, a Professor of Physiology at Toulouse, is best known for declaring in 1872 that 'Louis Pasteur's theory of germs is ridiculous fiction.' But stem cell science, built on imaginative yet rigorous assays by Till and McCulloch five decades ago, has already stood the test of time. Moving more of the science forward, taking it out of the research lab and into the hospital or clinic, is only a matter of time.

10

Little Fame, No Nobel

What do James Till and Ernest McCulloch have in common with fellow Canadians Norman Bethune and Wilder Penfield?

All four made enormous contributions to medical science. Bethune was a surgical innovator who invented and improved operating room instruments and developed mobile blood banks for wounded soldiers. Penfield founded the Montreal Neurological Institute and his research led to a far greater understanding of how the brain works, particularly for people with epilepsy. But not one of the four has won the highest honour in their field: the Nobel Prize for Physiology or Medicine. Only one Canadian has ever captured that prize: Sir Frederick Banting won it with Scotland's J.J.R. Macleod in 1923 for their joint work developing insulin to treat diabetes.

This, of course, depends on the definition of 'Canadian.' David H. Hubel was born in Windsor, Ontario, and grew up in Montreal, but his Nobel-winning research into how the brain processes visual information was done with 1981 co-winner Torsten Wiesel at Harvard Medical School. Charles B. Huggins, who won in 1966 for his discoveries in hormonal treatment of prostatic cancer, was born and raised in Halifax but worked in the United States. There is also British-born American geneticist Oliver Smithies, who shared the Nobel with Mario Capecchi and Sir Martin J. Evans for introducing specific gene modifications in 'knockout mice' by the use of embryonic stem cells. Smithies has a strong Canadian connection: a Briton who had worked in the United States, he was a University of Toronto researcher from 1954 until 1960, when, in part to ease his American wife's homesickness, he joined the genetics group at the University of Wisconsin. 'But I continued to collaborate with my Toronto friends to decipher the molecular/genetic basis of the protein differences found in plasma,' he says in his Nobel autobiography.[82]

But in terms of Canadians who did their best work in Canada, it has been a shutout for medical researchers since Banting despite the enormous accomplishments of Bethune, Penfield, and Till and McCulloch. But there is a big difference. Bethune, because of his much publicized work saving lives in the Spanish Civil War and in China, and Penfield, who developed the Montreal Procedure for seizure-relieving brain surgery, are revered in Canada and famous beyond our borders. Till and McCulloch? Not so much.

In 2004, the CBC, borrowing an idea from the BBC, launched *The Greatest Canadian* competition to highlight figures from Canada's past and present. More than 140,000 names were whittled down to a top 100 Canadians, whose order was decided by 1.2 million votes over the television program's run. The Top 100 list included medical innovators Banting (4) and his colleague Charles Best (77), and Norman Bethune (26), as well as pop culture figures like wrestler Bret Hart (39) and singer Avril Lavigne (40). In seventh place on the list was hockey commentator Don Cherry. Tommy Douglas, the father of medicare, took first.

The CBC followed up in 2007 with *The Greatest Canadian Invention*, which showcased fifty of Canada's top inventions. The winners included five-pin bowling and the Wonder Bra, as well as important medical discoveries such as the Cobalt bomb (11) and insulin (1).

Till and McCulloch and the discovery of stem cells made neither list.

David Naylor, President of the University of Toronto, sees three reasons why Till and McCulloch have been so overlooked in Canada and in Sweden.

'First, the public tends to focus on immediate applications,' Naylor explained in e-mail correspondence. 'Insulin could be used clinically more or less right away. It has taken decades for the full implications of their work to become clear.

'Second, Till and McCulloch have won every other prize in science, but, for reasons unknown, have not won a Nobel Prize despite multiple nominations. Those of us who have been involved in both nominations and selection processes for major scientific prizes understand that these matters are somewhat random and also highly political, but the public tends to focus still on the Nobel Prize.

'Third, the world lives by narratives. That helps to explain why Charles Best [Banting's assistant] has overshadowed J.J.R. Macleod, even though it was Macleod who won the Nobel Prize with Banting.

The narrative of insulin ended up focusing on the iconoclastic surgeon with his brilliant student protégé and friend. The story of Till and McCulloch simply has not been told often enough, perhaps because it has taken so long for their work to be appreciated.'

In terms of winning the Nobel, the time has now passed for McCulloch. Prizes aren't awarded posthumously unless a laureate passes away after the announcement of the award has been made. Till is still eligible to win, but whether one-half of a pioneering partnership will be honoured is anyone's guess.

There is precedent. As recently as 2010, Britain's Robert Edwards won the Nobel Prize for Physiology or Medicine for his work in *in vitro* fertilization. Edwards worked directly with gynecologist Patrick Steptoe, the man responsible for bringing the process to the clinic by using laparoscopy – a technique he pioneered. Steptoe died in 1988.

The fact that Till and McCulloch have not already won the Nobel remains a mystery to many – and not just Canadians who have wanted two of their own to triumph on the international stage. Stanford's Irving Weissman, perhaps the most important stem cell scientist currently working in the United States, routinely nominated Till and McCulloch for the Nobel – only to see them not be invited to the ceremony in Stockholm.

'I've been doing it since, I guess, the early to mid-1980s,' says Weissman. 'If I missed a year it was because they didn't ask me to nominate that year – you have to be asked to nominate people. They send out the nomination form only to a selected group of scientists.'

It all depends, says Weissman, on who reviews the nominations and what they take into consideration. 'You can hope. But nobody should gauge the success of their own career on whether they get that particular prize or not. There have been lots of times that people who made very important contributions didn't ever get the prize. Till and McCulloch are among that category.'

Weissman suggests that he has not been a lone voice crying out in the wilderness. 'Lots of people have nominated them.' Indeed, Weissman's compatriot David Scadden, who co-founded and co-directs the Harvard Stem Cell Institute and the Harvard University Department of Stem Cell and Regenerative Biology, can't fathom why they haven't won the big one.

'As one who hopes to stand on their shoulders, I love their work and they should win a Nobel Prize. Till and McCulloch clearly are giants. They clearly paved the way and made this whole field.'

The Nobel Prize recognizes outstanding achievements in physics, chemistry, physiology or medicine, literature, peace, and (since 1969) economics. Probably the most prestigious award a human being can receive, the Nobel is the legacy of Alfred Nobel, a Swedish chemist, engineer, and inventor, who amassed his fortune through many successful inventions – most notably dynamite.

The process for being awarded a Nobel is long, complex, and mysterious. To be nominated for the Nobel Prize in Physiology or Medicine, a candidate must have his or her name put forward by one of the roughly three thousand people invited by the Nobel Committee to act as nominators. Each September, the nominators are sent forms and are asked to submit their picks by 31 January. (Submissions are confidential.) The Nobel Committee then selects the preliminary candidates and consults with experts to assess the merits of each. Then in September, the Nobel Committee submits its final recommendations. The Nobel Laureates are chosen by a majority vote in the Nobel Assembly in October. The winners are announced that same month and receive their awards in December.

The Nobel organization does not discuss nominations. Requests for an interview were politely but firmly declined. 'We do not give interviews or answer any questions regarding who has/has not been nominated for the Nobel Prize.'

Nominations are supposed to be a closely guarded secret, but the biographies of Till and McCulloch produced by the University of Toronto Archives and Records Management indicate that they were nominated jointly in 2009.

'I won't discuss details, but they've been nominated a number of times,' says Alan Bernstein, former President of the Canadian Institutes of Health Research, who did his PhD with Till. He puts their lack of a Nobel down to bad luck and worse timing – and the fact that their earliest work appeared in niche journals instead of mainstream publications. 'They published their first two papers in *Radiation Research*. There wasn't a stem cell journal in those days, obviously. They were interested in the whole problem of radiation sensitivity during cancer therapy. So that was the origin of the work. But really, it should have been in *Nature* or *Science* ... which I think is important. I think it contributed to the downplay: nobody in developmental biology or stem cells, whatever, would have read *Radiation Research*. So it was buried for a long time. And they never used the words "stem cells." Jim, in particular, was a real stickler for operational definitions. "That's what science is," as he would say. So they called it colony-forming units in the spleen and the broader world out there never really caught on to what they were doing.'

That's why, Bernstein says, Till and McCulloch have remained relatively unknown.

'Time has passed them by to some extent, unfortunately. The [1998] discovery of human embryonic stem cells has captivated the world and people are very excited about human embryonic stem cells, but that's a completely different field than hematopoietic stem cells. There's a disconnect between the two fields. The basic context and definition and criteria for what you call stem cells were established by Till and McCulloch. Whether everybody working on embryonic stem cells knows this, I'm not sure. I'm sure a lot of people just don't appreciate the contributions that Till and McCulloch made. You just take it for granted. You don't think, "Well, these are the two guys that figured it out."'

Till and McCulloch have not gone without honours. In 1969 they won the Gairdner Award, Canada's top prize for health research. They won the 2005 Albert Lasker Award for Basic Medical Research for what the Lasker Foundation called 'ingenious experiments that first identified a stem cell – the blood-forming stem cell – which set the stage for all current research on adult and embryonic stem cells.' Since 1945, the Lasker has been the ultimate accolade for health research in North America and is often the precursor to winning the big one: eighty Lasker Laureates have received the Nobel Prize, including twenty-eight in the past two decades.[83]

The possibility of winning a Nobel Prize is plainly not something that keeps Jim Till up at night composing potential acceptance speeches. In the wake of the Lasker win, when he was asked for his thoughts on winning a Nobel, he responded in his typical low-key style. 'I can only respond that this is not why we did this kind of work,' he told the *Toronto Star*.[84] 'This is not why I went into science. Were it to happen – I mean I have no idea – I would feel the same way as I do about the Lasker: it would be great for science in Canada in general and stem cell science in particular. Again, because the field is quite controversial, it hasn't had that much recognition yet. My hope is that it will get a lot more. And I'm hoping that we're the beginning of a trend.'

Asked whether Canadians ought to know as much about Till and McCulloch as they do about Banting and Best, McCulloch responded in his characteristic wry style. 'When we're dead. Privacy to me is very important.'

McCulloch and Till have both stressed they were only ever interested in science for the sake of science – for gathering knowledge and seeing where things lead. Being prize-winning science celebrities was never part of the plan. 'I think actually those who seek celebrity risk compromising themselves in terms of their science,' Till said in the *Star* article. 'It's very tough to produce creative work on schedule. That's what you have to do in order to maintain a celebrity status. That kind of game is not for me. It never was.'

There has been some conjecture that the 2007 breakthrough discovery by Japan's Shinya Yamanaka, which showed that induced pluripotent stem (iPS) cells can be created from human adult skin tissue, has presented an opportunity to correct what many see as an oversight.

Lorne Tyrrell, former Dean of the Faculty of Medicine and Dentistry at the University of Alberta, suggests that the Till and McCulloch oversight could be corrected if – more likely when – the iPS cell discovery is honoured with a Nobel.

'The Nobel Prize is usually given to a discovery that has broad impact,' says Tyrrell. 'Yamanaka has altered some of the problems of the source of stem cells, allowing for the development of pluripotent stem cells from normal tissue. What has always been there is potential, tantalizing potential, never fully captured. Now that work [by Yamanaka] has allowed it to be moved very rapidly forward. I think there is a very good chance it will happen. I have no inside information, but look at regenerative medicine and how important it's becoming – and it's really based on those [Till and McCulloch] discoveries.'

There is more at stake than individual honour. 'It would be critically important,' says Tyrrell. 'Medical research in Canada needs the kind of boost a Nobel victory would provide. Canada puts a lot of research money into medical research and there have been a number of excellent Canadian discoveries. It would be a really important signal to the Canadian government and Canadians that Canada is doing internationally competitive work.'

Guy Sauvageau, the Founding Scientific Director and CEO of the Institute for Research in Immunology and Cancer at the University of Montreal, agrees. 'If you look at Canada, we have a number of Nobel Laureates, but the majority of them were awarded when the winners were outside of Canada. It's not for the work that they did in Canada, but because they were born Canadian. I think we're probably one of the worst if not the worst country in this area [physiology or medicine]. I was hoping that we would get one from this, because I think this is a true Canadian finding and it is in an area where Canada has been a leading country in the world.'

Along with Bethune and Penfield, Till and McCulloch are not the only Canadians to have their outstanding work overlooked by the Nobel Committee. In 1931, Frederick Tisdall, Theodore Drake, and Alan Brown, working out of the University of Toronto, introduced Pablum, a nutritional breakthrough that helped prevent rickets in infants.

Like Till and McCulloch, Charles Philippe Leblond was a Gairdner winner and member of the Canadian Medical Hall of Fame. Born in France in 1910, he came to McGill University in 1941 and over many years developed autoradiography, a technique for visualizing radioactively labelled tissue or cells. Leblond died in Montreal in 2007, having never won a Nobel.

The lack of Canadian Nobels in medical research might reflect 'a Canadian problem,' suggests Oxford University's Sir John Bell. 'Canadians are, by nature, not very pushy or flashy. As a result they often don't get the public attention that they deserve. So I would say that outside of Canada there are probably quite a large number of biomedical scientists who don't recognize the contribution that Till and McCulloch made.'

And unlike the United States, Bell says, Canada doesn't go full-throttle to promote its true patriot scientific sons and daughters. 'I don't know if you've ever seen the machines that they throw into force in big American universities to promote their own internal people. I've never seen anything equivalent to it in the United Kingdom or in Canada. We tend to be slightly more modest and assume that if [Nobel] committees are thinking about it they'll obviously get there in the end. The truth is that doesn't actually happen.'

National pride aside, the work done by Till and McCulloch deserves the biggest prize in medical research. 'Without question,' says Michael Rudnicki, Scientific Director of the Canadian Stem Cell Network. 'Given the current status of stem cell research and regenerative medicine – their work paved the way for all that – why they haven't received that, I really have no idea. In my mind, there is no one that comes close to those two and their contributions.'

As the University of Toronto's Naylor noted, the lack of a Nobel has kept Till and McCulloch's story from being told and retold to ordinary Canadians. They have remained relatively unknown, especially when compared to actors, rock stars, and hockey players.

'They are known in the stem cell world internationally for their contributions,' says Gordon Keller, Director of the McEwen Centre for Regenerative Medicine. 'But that's true for many places: you often don't know what's happening in your backyard.'

Conclusion

While describing the protagonist of his satiric novel *Solar*, the acclaimed British novelist Ian McEwan captures the sense of pure awe that perfectly executed science can evoke:

> At the age of twenty-one he had read in wonder the Dirac Equation of 1928 in its full form, predicting the spin of an electron. A thing of pure beauty, that equation, one of the greatest intellectual feats ever performed, correctly demanding of nature the existence of antiparticles and placing before the young reader the wide horizons of the 'Dirac sea.'[85]

While McEwan was writing about one of the pivotal publications in modern theoretical physics, his words could easily be adapted to another thing of pure beauty: the 1961 *Radiation Research* paper by James Edgar Till and Ernest Armstrong McCulloch. Throughout the interviews conducted for this book, scientists routinely referred to the work as 'elegant' and 'powerful.' Others favoured terms like 'robust' and 'rigorous.' The word 'seminal' also came up frequently, and with good reason. The discovery of hematopoietic stem cells, which set in place the footings for what would become stem cell science and regenerative medicine, ranks alongside the Paul Dirac epistle that prepared the ground for quantum mechanics. Their subsequent work poured the foundations that rested on those footings.

'It's a very significant inflection point in our understanding of that particular bit of biology,' says Sir John Bell, the Regius Chair of Medicine at Oxford University. 'Today it's already tied into immunological and hematological diseases, but I suspect it will have much wider applications as other developments in tissue regeneration come into play. It basically underpins almost everything that we now know about development. It's not the only component, obviously. There's the influence of various growth factors ... the evolution of any particular lineage, the development of induced pluripotent stem cells, all those things have added substantially to our understanding of the biology and our approaches to manipulate it. But if you had to track it back to the conceptual recognition of single cell populations that self-renew and lead to the creation of specific differentiated cells, then that's Till and McCulloch.'

The early work that Till and McCulloch scribbled out in pencil on graph paper notebooks and punched in on manual typewriters with carbon-paper copies has stood the test of time and continues to be current in a high-speed Internet, computer-in-your-pocket universe.

'Till and McCulloch were the first to apply mathematical modelling to stem cells,' says Peter Zandstra of the University of Toronto's Institute of Biomaterials and Biomedical Engineering. 'Those models basically set up the last fifty years of stem cell research. What is really exciting is that we are now in a wonderful position to go back into this interdisciplinary area of using mathematical modelling and systems biology to reveal new layers of control in stem cell fate decisions and get new information about how the environment in the body controls stem cell development.'

That their work endures and continues to be both revered and relevant is due to two things: the imagination involved in envisioning the creation of cells, and the rigour brought to the task of capturing that crucial biological function. The work is infused with genius and steeped in tenacity. Many assume that McCulloch was the source of that intellectual sparkle while Till did the yeoman service of supplying the steadfastness required to verify and validate the findings. The overly modest Till has added credence to this theory by suggesting he 'rode Ernest's coattails' while they were conducting their superior science. It is a compelling way to look at the partnership, almost as if they were a songwriting team in which one wrote the unforgettable melodies while the other found the right words to match, but it does neither man full justice.

'Society often tries to put people into boxes that describe their personalities as if this person was this type and that person was that type and that's why they worked well together,' says Connie Eaves, the now world-renowned cancer researcher, who as a newly minted PhD showed up on Dr McCulloch's OCI office doorstep in 1970 seven months pregnant and ready to get to work.

'There's no question that they had different training and different perspectives. Jim brought a knowledge of physics and math and statistics, had it at his fingertips, and had a way of thinking that Bunny didn't have. And Bunny brought knowledge of human disease, and physiology and complexity of dealing with cells that Jim did not have. But, having said that, they then merged those abilities to tackle problems in a way that when two people work well together, they know how to work well together. It's not so easy or even useful to stereotype them as this is the "this" person, and that is the "that" person.

'It's true in writing manuscripts, that Bunny would often come up with phraseologies that were able to express complex ideas in a compelling way that was highly readable. That was a significant talent that he had. And Jim was also able to think of how to draw a diagram or create a way of presenting data that conveyed the message in a simplified, bolder fashion because that's what elements would come out. But I think it would be a big mistake to stereotype them.'

Indeed, either man was capable of great imagination and astounding attention to detail. McCulloch might have been an idea-a-minute, big-picture thinker, but his first reaction upon seeing the bumps on the mouse spleens on that Sunday in 1960 was not to marvel at their beauty, but to count them. To plot the results on a graph. To see if the numbers added up. And in his application of a stochastic approach to statistics to explain variations within the colony-forming units, Till displayed a facility for grand thinking that most scientists can only hope to achieve.

Alan Bernstein, who learned how to do science at Till's knee, says that while each man certainly had his particular strengths, either could do whatever needed to be done to move the science forward.

'The natural personalities were essential to being in that relationship. Jim became the roots, the solid guy who had everything under control, and Bun became more, well, was allowed to become the more out-of-the-box thinker because Jim would bring him down to earth. But like in any partnership or relationship, if one person is A, the other person has to be not A to balance it a little bit. When I travel with my wife, if I'm worried about not catching a flight, she'll be the one that's calm. And if she's worried, I'm the one that's calm.'

So while it is attractive to apply a head-in-the-clouds label to McCulloch and a feet-on-the-ground tag to Till, it isn't entirely accurate. Like all myths, it resonates with truth but does not capture reality. Labels and tags are too limiting. McCulloch was more than a dreamer and Till was much more than a wizard with numbers.

'McCulloch was the one that had ideas every two minutes and Jim was the one that really helped design the rigorous experiments to make sure the data were analysed correctly,' says Bob Phillips, another OCI alumnus who did great work in cancer research. 'But the whole concept of stochastic model and stem cells, that was all Jim Till. And that's had a big impact on the field. I remember sitting in meetings when we would be discussing findings from experiments and certainly Jim would contribute a lot of ideas and concepts. It's just that McCulloch was the dominant brainstormer.'

Certainly, though, Till, with his easygoing Prairie-boy affability, and McCulloch, with his upper-crust Ontario formality, evoked very different responses from the people who worked alongside them and for them. As a result, each seemed to attract his own kind of acolyte.

McCulloch bewildered some with his fondness for dropping arcane references into scientific discussions. 'He was a very imposing figure because of his quick mind and to engage with him in an intellectual discussion was a humbling experience,' says a McCulloch colleague from the early days at the OCI.

McCulloch definitely could be intellectually intimidating. Engaging in a conversation with him was akin to walking into a windstorm: he was a force that could come at you from a number of directions. He could be wonderfully warm and charming. He could be acerbic, delivering criticism that was withering. Chewing on his piece of chalk, he could be inscrutable. He could demand great things and then not say thanks upon their delivery. Then, later, he would offer an invitation to his cottage. He fostered an almost cult-like loyalty among many of those who worked closely with him. Many stayed friends with him for life.

'I organized a birthday party for him when he turned eighty,' says Tak Mak, a self-admitted member of the 'McCulloch cult' of OCI-schooled researchers whose members are now at work across Canada and around the world. 'I invited all his closest and best friends to come and they all came. I had a talk with him that night and I had never felt so content and complete, just the way he looked at me, that I'd done this for him. He never tells you his real feelings. But it is understood.'

For his part, McCulloch said he intimidated no one and was just one of a talented group of people doing innovative work at the OCI. In an interview for this book a few months before his death, McCulloch worried about being mythologized. 'I hope you won't make too big a thing,' he said. He maintained he wasn't all that well read. 'My knowledge of history is pretty weak, I've just finished reading a book on the Second World War which showed me how little I knew during it, how little I appreciated what was going on.'

He took satisfaction in the fact that his friendship with Till lasted long after their science partnership gave way to each man pursuing his own path. 'One of the things I'm happiest about is that after all these years later, we're very good friends.'[86]

Till remains a firm-handshake, hearty-laugh individual who looks like he just walked in out of a wheat field. He is easy to approach and less likely to confuse. But he too is not without the ability to intimidate, with a piercing stare that locks on a listener while his mind calculates the value of what's being said. He can be stunningly frank and disarmingly honest. One scientist told of Till commenting, 'Well, I wouldn't do it,' about an experiment he was about to embark on, 'but if you think it's a good idea, then go ahead.' Till was a hands-off mentor who, unlike his partner, didn't jump in with suggestions and interventions. He was, and remains, an excellent sounding board, someone to bounce ideas off of, work problems out with. Someone who will give a straight answer. But as no-nonsense as he is, he was able to work closely with his sometimes maddeningly off-the-wall collaborator.

'We had absolute trust in each other,' says Till. 'When you have that personal trust, you can basically say anything to each other, right or wrong, crazy or not. You can just explore and that's what we could do as I see it. It was perfect. I can only talk about my view of Ernest McCulloch and I could say anything to him. If I didn't like it, I'd say so and why. If he did like it, he'd say so and why. I had never any doubt about his integrity in terms of dealing with our entire collaboration.'

Their first paper, a 1960 examination of the radiation sensitivity of normal mouse bone marrow cells, hinted at what was to come.[87] A year later, they introduced the world to colony-forming units, proving the existence of stem cells.[88]

'If it had stopped there – if that was the only experiment they had published – it would have been enough to give them many prizes,' says Stanford's stem cell giant Irving Weissman. 'But they had four papers that defined our field.'[89]

In 1963, they fortified their stem cell proof by demonstrating the clonal nature of the spleen colonies – tracking the origins of blood to a single cell.[90] They expanded on it further that year, with the help of geneticist Lou Siminovitch, by explaining the distribution of the colony-forming cells in spleen colonies.[91] The Till-led 1964 paper on the stochastic model of stem cell proliferation became required reading on the randomness involved in how stem cells develop.[92] As late as 1980 they were co-authoring ground-breaking papers that explained blood-based stem cell proliferation.[93]

While their work was not directly responsible for the development of bone marrow transplantation – Nobel Laureate E. Donnall Thomas was already hard at work on it in the United States when Till and McCulloch were just embarking on their partnership – their findings provided the theoretical underpinning to support it. And their work is directly responsible for the beginning of successful bone marrow transplantation programs in Canada.

The legacy they have left is far more than a handful of papers that defined stem cell science. At laboratories and clinics across Canada and around the world, researchers and clinicians have been influenced, directly or indirectly, by the 'OCI culture' of imaginative thinking and exacting rigour that Harold Johns and Arthur Ham insisted upon and that Till and McCulloch absorbed and passed on to the following generations. 'I actually take some pride in that,' says Till. I take more pride in that than I do in the original observations, which were, well, Ernest made the original observations of the bumps on the spleens of these mice. He deserves the kudos for that.'[94]

Those scientists of whom Till is so proud are now pushing back the limits of knowledge about cancer and a number of degenerative diseases. They are thinking big, but also paying acute attention to the molecularly tiny details that reveal the truth. They are carrying on in the Till and McCulloch tradition that demands equal parts passion and patience, creativity and critical thinking, dreams and due diligence.

Notes

1 Ernest A. McCulloch, *The Ontario Cancer Institute: Success and Reverses at Sherbourne Street* (Montreal and Kingston: McGill-Queen's University Press, 2003), 47.

2 Louis Pasteur, 'Inaugural lecture,' University of Lille, 7 December 1854.

3 'Canadiens' Richard, 29, Quits Hockey,' *Chicago Daily Tribune*, 16 September 1960, E1.

4 David Spurgeon, 'Scientists Humbled as Human Knowledge Grows,' *The Globe and Mail*, 1 January 1960, 3.

5 George Bain, 'Partners in Aid Sought by U.S.,' *The Globe and Mail*, 1 January 1960, 3.

6 Salk Institute for Biological Studies, 'About Jonas Salk,' accessed 26 September 2010. http://www.salk.edu/about/jonas_salk.html.

7 Ivan Noble, '"Secret of Life" Discovery Turns 50,' *BBC News Online*, 27 February 2003, accessed 26 September 2010. http://news.bbc.co.uk/2/hi/science/nature/2804545.stm.

8 McCulloch, *The Ontario Cancer Institute*, 3.

9 CBC Digital Archives, 'Debut of the Cobalt Bomb,' accessed 26 September 2010. http://archives.cbc.ca/science_technology/natural_science/clips/1855.

10 Canada Science and Technology Museum, 'Artifact Spotlight,' accessed 26 September 2010. http://www.sciencetech.technomuses.ca/english/collection/artifact-spotlight.cfm.

11 Canadian Nuclear Association, 'The Cobalt-60 Therapy Unit,' accessed 26 September 2010. http://www.cna.ca/curriculum/cna_nuc_tech/cobalt60-eng.asp?bc=Cobalt-60%20Therapy%20Unit&pid=Cobalt-60%20Therapy%20Unit.

12 Ed Willett, 'Sask. First to Make "Cobalt bomb,"' *The Leader-Post* (Regina), 28 September 2006, A6.

13 Alison Kraft, 'Manhattan Transfer: Lethal Radiation, Bone Marrow Transplantation, and the Birth of Stem Cell Biology, c. 1942–1961,' *Historical Studies in the Natural Sciences* 39 (2009): 181–218 at 173.
14 Carolyn Abraham, 'Scientist Was Pioneer in Stem Cell Research,' *The Globe and Mail*, 29 January 2011, S11.
15 McCulloch, *The Ontario Cancer Institute*, 18.
16 Ibid., 67.
17 Lou Siminovitch, *Reflections on a Life in Science* (Toronto: L. Siminovitch, 2003), 77.
18 Miguel Ramalho-Santos and Holger Willenbring, 'On the Origin of the Term "Stem Cell,"' *Cell Stem Cell* 1 (2007): 35–8, accessed 17 March 2011. http://www.cell.com/cell-stem-cell/fulltext/S1934-5909(07)00019-7.
19 Kraft, 'Manhattan Transfer,' 200.
20 McCulloch, *The Ontario Cancer Institute*, 55.
21 D.H. Cowan, 'Vera Peters and the Curability of Hodgkin Disease,' *Current Oncology* 15 (October 2008): 206–10, accessed 29 March 2011. http://www.ncbi.nlm.nih.gov/pmc/articles/PMC2582517.
22 McCulloch, *The Ontario Cancer Institute*, 55.
23 John J. Trentin, 'Determination of Bone Marrow Stem Cell Differentiation by Stromal Hemopoietic Inductive Microenvironments,' *American Journal of Pathology* 65 (1971): 621–8.
24 D.W.H. Barnes, E.P. Evans, C.E. Ford, and B.J. West, 'Spleen Colonies in Mice: Karyotypic Evidence of Multiple Colonies from Single Cells,' *Nature* 219 (1968): 518–20.
25 McCulloch, *The Ontario Cancer Institute*, 55.
26 Evelyn Strauss, 'The Lasker Foundation: Albert Lasker Basic Research Award: Award Description,' Lasker Foundation, accessed 26 September 2010. http://www.laskerfoundation.org/awards/2005_b_description.htm.
27 McCulloch, *The Ontario Cancer Institute*, 7.
28 S. Spence Meighan and H.A. Bean, 'Attempted Homotransplantation of Bone Marrow in a Patient with Leukæmia,' Cases Studies, *Canadian Medical Association Journal* 78, no. 1 (1 June 1958): 858–62.
29 L.J. Kleinsmith and G.B. Pierce. 'Multipotentiality of Single Embryonal Carcinoma Cells,' *Cancer Research* 24 (1964): 1544–51.
30 Rick Weiss, 'A Crucial Human Cell Isolated, Multiplied,' *Washington Post*, 6 November 1998, A1, accessed 28 March 2011. http://www.washingtonpost.com/wp-srv/national/cell110698.htm.
31 Carolyn Abraham, 'Citizenship Costs Canadian Top Stem Cell Post,' *The Globe and Mail*, 4 December 2010, A8.
32 Siminovitch, *Reflections on a Life in Science*, 158.

33 Y. Yanagi, Y. Yoshikai, K. Leggett, S.P. Clark, I. Aleksander, and T.W. Mak, 'A Human T Cell-Specific cDNA Clone Encodes a Protein Having Extensive Homology to Immunoglobulin Chains,' *Nature* 308 (1984): 145–9.

34 McCulloch, *The Ontario Cancer Institute*, 135.

35 'The Hottest Papers of 1998–99,' *ScienceWatch*, March–April 2000, accessed 22 March 2011. http://archive.sciencewatch.com/march-april2000/sw_march-april2000_page1.htm.

36 McCulloch, *The Ontario Cancer Institute*, 137–8.

37 M. Mayer and J.E. Till, 'The Internet: A Modern Pandora's Box?' *Quality of Life Research* 5 (1996): 568–71.

38 Mike King, 'Leukemia Linked to Two Genes,' *The Gazette* (Montreal), 13 May 2003, A1.

39 'Researchers Claim Stem Cell Victory,' *The Gazette* (Montreal), 17 April 2009, A6.

40 B.A. Reynolds and S. Weiss, 'Generation of Neurons and Astrocytes from Isolated Cells of the Adult Mammalian Central Nervous System,' *Science* 255 (1992): 1707–10.

41 Monya Baker, 'John Dick: Careful Assays for Cancer Stem Cells,' *Nature.com*, 26 March 2009, accessed 11 November 2010. http://www.nature.com/stemcells/2009/0903/090326/full/stemcells.2009.47.html.

42 John E. Dick, 'Stem Cell Concepts Renew Cancer Research,' *Blood* 112 (2008): 4793–807.

43 Jeffrey M. Perkel, 'Colon Cancer Stem Cells Identified,' *The Scientist*, 20 November 2006, accessed 11 November 2010. http://www.the-scientist.com/news/display/36646.

44 J. Stingl, P. Eirew, I. Ricketson, M. Shackleton, F. Vaillant, D. Choi, H.I. Li, and C.J. Eaves, 'Purification and Unique Properties of Mammary Epithelial Stem Cells,' *Nature* 439 (2006): 993–7.

45 G.Q. Daley, L. Ahrlund Richter, J.M. Auerbach, N. Benvenisty, R.A. Charo, G. Chen, H.K. Deng, L.S. Goldstein, K.L. Hudson, I. Hyun, S.C. Junn, J. Love, E.H. Lee, A. McLaren, C.L. Mummery, N. Nakatsuji, C. Racowsky, H. Rooke, J. Rossant, H.R. Schöler, J.H. Solbakk, P. Taylor, A.O. Trounson, I.L. Weissman, I. Wilmut, J. Yu, and L. Zoloth, 'Ethics: The ISSCR Guidelines for Human Embryonic Stem Cell Research,' *Science* 315 (2007): 603–4.

46 Margaret Munro, 'Embryo Research Stirs Hope Fear,' *Times Colonist* (Victoria), 6 October 2005, A5.

47 Tom Spears, 'Toronto Hospital Makes Stem Cell Breakthrough,' *Kingston Whig-Standard*, 9 June 2005, 20.

48 Mount Sinai Hospital, 'Dr Andras Nagy makes *Scientific American* Top 10 Honor Roll,' accessed 24 March 2011. http://www.mountsinai.on.ca/

about_us/news/2009/dr-andras-nagy-makes-scientific-american-top-10-honor-roll.

49 J.G. Toma, M Akhavan., K.J.L. Fernandes, M.P. Fortier, F. Barnabé-Heider, A. Sadikot, D.R. Kaplan, and F.D. Miller, 'Isolation of Multipotent Adult Stem Cells from the Dermis of Mammalian Skin,' *Nature Cell Biology* 3 (2001): 778–84.

50 Ontario Consultants on Religious Tolerance, 'Stem Cell Research: All Viewpoints,' accessed 28 September 2010. http://www.religioustolerance.org/res_stem.htm.

51 CNN, 'Transcript: Pope John Paul II,' accessed 28 September 2010. http://transcripts.cnn.com/2001/WORLD/europe/07/23/bush.pope.

52 LeRoy Walters, 'Human Embryonic Stem Cell Research: An Intercultural Perspective,' *Kennedy Institute of Ethics Journal* 14 (2004): 3–38.

53 'Dobson Likened Embryonic Stem Cell Research to Nazi Experiments,' *Media Matters for America*, 3 August 2005, accessed 28 September 2010. http://mediamatters.org/mmtv/200508030007.

54 'Bill C-56: An Act Respecting Assisted Human Reproduction,' Government of Canada, 27 May 2002, accessed 28 September 2010. http://dsp-psd.pwgsc.gc.ca/Collection-R/LoPBdP/LS/371/371c56-e.htm#%284%29.

55 Françoise Baylis, 'Betwixt and Between Human Stem Cell Guidelines and Legislation,' *Health Law Review* 11 (2002): 44–50.

56 'Bill C-56.'

57 'Bill C-13, Assisted Human Reproduction Act,' Parliament of Canada, 10 October 2002, accessed 28 September 2010. http://www2.parl.gc.ca/Sites/LOP/LegislativeSummaries/Bills_ls.asp?lang=E&Parl=37&Ses=2&ls=C13&source=Bills_House_Government.

58 Timothy Caulfield, 'Bill C-13: The Assisted Human Reproduction Act: Examining the Arguments against a Regulatory Approach,' *Health Law Review* 11 (2002): 20–5.

59 Kristen Philipkoski, 'Canada Closes Door on Cloning,' *Wired*, 17 March 2004, accessed 28 September 2010. http://www.wired.com/medtech/health/news/2004/03/62695.

60 'President George W. Bush's Address on Stem Cell Research,' *CNN.com*, 9 August 2001, accessed 28 September 2010. http://edition.cnn.com/2001/ALLPOLITICS/08/09/bush.transcript/index.html.

61 Brandon Keim, 'With Bush Ban Gone, Stem Cell Research Will Proliferate,' *Wired*, 9 March 2009, accessed 28 September 2010. http://www.wired.com/wiredscience/2009/03/obamastemcells.

62 Gardiner Harris, 'U.S. Judge Rules Against Obama's Stem Cell Policy,' *New York Times*, 24 August 2010, accessed 28 September 2010. http://www.nytimes.com/2010/08/24/health/policy/24stem.html?hp.

63 Philipkoski, 'Canada Closes Door on Cloning.'

64 Pew Forum on Religion and Public Life, 'Stem Cell Research Around the World,' accessed 28 September 2010. http://pewforum.org/Science-and-Bioethics/Stem-Cell-Research-Around-the-World.aspx.

65 Ibid.

66 'MMR-Row Doctor Failed in His Duties,' *Yorkshire Evening Post*, 28 January 2010, accessed 28 September 2010. http://www.yorkshireeveningpost.co.uk/news/BREAKING-MMR-expert-failed-in.6024127.jp.

67 Jeffrey Kluger, 'Jenny McCarthy on Autism and Vaccines,' *Time Magazine*, 1 April 2009, accessed 11 November 2010. http://www.time.com/time/health/article/0,8599,1888718,00.html.

68 Sam Lister, 'Steep Rise in Measles Cases Blamed on MMR Scare,' *The Times of London*, 6 February 2009, accessed 11 November 2010. http://www.timesonline.co.uk/tol/life_and_style/health/child_health/article5674974.ece.

69 'Health Officials Warn Public about Increased Risk of Measles,' *City News Toronto*, 4 April 2008, accessed 28 September 2010. http://www.citytv.com/toronto/citynews/life/health/article/22085-health-officials-warn-public-about-increased-risk-of-measles.

70 Agence France-Presse, 'UK Climate Scientists Cleared of Dishonesty,' *Nanaimo Daily News*, 8 July 2010, accessed 28 June 2011. http://www2.canada.com/nanaimodailynews/news/nation/story.html?id=cb203228-3bae-4760-9aaa-4c5031d550ac.

71 Mike DeSouza and Sheldon Alberts, 'Caution over Climate Change "Wise": Bernier,' *National Post*, 25 February 2010, A5.

72 Megan Ogilvie, 'Stem Cell Breakthrough "Too Simple,"' *Toronto Star*, 30 October 2009, GT3.

73 Joseph Hall, 'McMaster Breakthrough Raises Transfusion Hopes,' *Toronto Star*, 8 November 2010, A3.

74 Stem Cell Network, 'Canadian Innovations in Stem Cell Therapeutics,' *Northern Lights*, Summer 2009, 13.

75 Lori P. Knowles, 'Stem Cell Hype and the Dangers of Stem Cell "Tourism,"' *Stem Cell Network White Papers*, accessed 22 October 2010. http://www.stemcellnetwork.ca/uploads/File/whitepapers/Stem-Cell-Hype.pdf.

76 GlaxoSmithKline, 'Largest Efficacy Trial of Cervical Cancer Vaccine Showed Cervarix™ Protects Against Five Most Common Cancer Causing Virus Types,' *GSK Media Release*, 7 July 2009, accessed 22 October 2010. http://www.gsk.ca/english/html/media-centre/docs-pdf/Cervarix_008_Lancet_Jul_7_2009.pdf.

77 National Institutes of Health, 'Stem Cells and Diseases,' accessed 22 October 2010. http://stemcells.nih.gov/info/health.asp.

78 U.S. National Institutes of Health. 'Search of: Stem Cells – List Results – Clinical Trials.gov,' accessed 21 January 2011. http://clinicaltrials.gov/search/term=stem+cells?term=stem+cells.

79 T. Lapidot, C. Sirard, J. Vormoor, F. Pflumio, T. Hoang, J. Caceres-Cortes, M. Minden, B. Patterson, M. Caligiuri, and J.E. Dick, 'A Cell Initiating Human Acute Myeloid Leukaemia after Transplantation into SCID Mice,' *Nature* 367 (1994): 645–8.

80 Sean J. Morrison, 'Efficient Tumour Formation by Single Human Melanoma Cells,' *Nature* 456 (2008): 593–8.

81 Sean J. Morrison, 'Mechanisms That Regulate Stem Cell Function,' *Howard Hughes Medical Institute*, accessed 28 September 2010. http://www.hhmi.org/research/investigators/morrison.html.

82 Oliver Smithies, 'Autobiography,' Nobelprize.org, accessed 17 March. http://nobelprize.org/nobel_prizes/medicine/laureates/2007/smithies.html.

83 The Lasker Foundation website, accessed 27 June 2011. http://www.laskerfoundation.org/awards/index.htm.

84 Joe Sornberger, 'T.O. Stem Cell Pioneers Win "America's Nobel,"' *Toronto Star*, 8 September 2005, A8.

85 Ian McEwan, *Solar* (Toronto: Knopf Canada, 2010), 25.

86 Joe Sornberger, 'Canadians Till and McCulloch Proved the Existence of Stem Cells,' *Stem Cell Network News Magazine* 3, no. 1 (1960): 7.

87 E.A. McCulloch and J.E. Till, 'The Radiation Sensitivity of Normal Mouse Bone Marrow Cells, Determined by Quantitative Marrow Transplantation into Irradiated Mice,' *Radiation Research* 13 (1960): 115–25.

88 J.E Till and E.A. McCulloch, 'A Direct Measurement of the Radiation Sensitivity of Normal Mouse Bone Marrow Cells,' *Radiation Research* 14 (1961): 213–22.

89 Sornberger, 'Canadians Till and McCulloch,' 3.

90 A.J. Becker, E.A. McCulloch, and J.E. Till, 'Cytological Demonstration of the Clonal Nature of Spleen Colonies Derived from Transplanted Mouse Marrow Cells,' *Nature* 197 (1963): 452–54.

91 L. Siminovitch, E.A. McCulloch, and J.E. Till, 'The Distribution of Colony-Forming Cells among Spleen Colonies,' *Journal of Cellular and Comparative Physiology* 62 (1963): 327–36.

92 J.E. Till, E.A. McCulloch, and L. Siminovitch, 'A Stochastic Model of Stem Cell Proliferation, Based on the Growth of Spleen Colony-Forming Cells,' *Proceedings of the National Academy of Sciences of the U.S.A.* 51 (1964): 29–36.

93 J.E. Till and E.A. McCulloch, 'Hemopoietic Stem Cell Differentiation,' *Biochimica et Biophysica Acta* 605 (1980): 431–59.

94 Sornberger, 'Canadians Till and McCulloch,' 7.

Index

Abu-Zahra, Hakam, 57
advanced cell technology, 98
Advanced Medical Discovery Institute, 54
Ali, Muhammad (Clay, Cassius), 13
Amato, Dominick, 57
Amgen Institute, 54
Atkins, Harry, 107–10, 112–14
Atwood, Margaret, 14
Austin Motor Company, 14
Aye, Bertie, 57

Bain, George, 15
Banting, Sir Frederick, 4, 126–7, 130
Banting Institute, 25
Barnes, D.W.H., 40
Beatles, The, 13
Becker, Andy, 26, 34, 36–7
Behie, Leo, 120
Bell, Sir John, 42–3, 124, 132, 133–4
Bergsagel, Daniel, 57
Bernier, Maxime, 91
Bernstein, Alan, 43–4, 49–54, 61, 71, 74–6, 100, 129–30, 135
Best, Charles, 4, 127, 130
Bethune, Norman, 126–7, 131
Bhatia, Mick, 38, 92
Boshkung Lake retreats, 29
Boveri, Theodor, 31
Boyd, Norman, 64
Brown, Alan, 132
Bruce, Robert, 28–9, 58
Bush, George W., 86–7, 89

California Institute for Regenerative Medicine, 50, 102
Campbell Family Institute for Breast Cancer Research, 55
Canadian Institutes of Health Research, 29, 43, 50, 64, 88, 129
Cancer Stem Cell Consortium, 55, 102
Capecchi, Mario R., 44, 126
Caulfield, Timothy, 87–9, 91
Checker, Chubby, 13
Cherry, Don, 127
Cinader, Bernhard, 28
Clarke, Michael, 100–1
Clarysse, Albert, 57
Cobalt bomb, 17–18, 24, 28, 127
Congdon, Charles, 37
Connery, Sean, 13
Cowan, Don, 57
Crick, Francis, 16

Cunningham, Alastair, 61–3
Curie, Marie, 17

Darte, John, 41–2, 57
Davis, Mark, 53
Dick, John, 4, 70–2, 100–4, 119
Diefenbaker, John G., 12
Dirac, Paul, 133
Dirks, Peter, 100–2, 104
Dobson, James, 86–7
Douglas, Tommy, 127
Drake, Theodore, 132
Dykstra, Brad, 80–1

Eaves, Allen, 58–60, 119–20
Eaves, Connie, 4, 58–9, 66, 72–4, 80, 134–5
Edwards, Robert, 128
Evans, Sir Martin J., 44, 126

Fleming, Alexander, 10
Food and Drug Administration, 96–7
Ford, Charles, 37
Fox, Michael J., 124
Fred Hutchinson Cancer Research Center, 41
Freedman, Mark, 108–10, 112–14
Frost, Leslie, 18
Fuerst, Clarence, 28

Gable, Clark, 13
Ganoza, Clelia, 34
Geron Corporation, 98
Goodyear, Charles, 10
Graham, Angus, 25

Haeckel, Ernst, 31
Ham, Arthur, 20, 28, 138
Hansen, Rick, 122–4
Hart, Bret, 127
Hasselback, Richard, 57
Hassell, John, 100–2, 104
Herzenberg, Leon, 39
Hitchcock, Alfred, 13
Hoffer, Abram, 62
Hubel, David H., 126
Huggins, Charles B., 126
Humphries, Keith, 73

International Society for Stem Cell Research, 78
Iscove, Norman, 57, 107, 114

Jacobson, Leon O., 17, 32
John Paul II, Pope, 86–7, 89
Johns, Harold, 17, 20–1, 24–5, 28–9, 138

Kallman, Robert, 35
Keating, Armand, 58
Keller, Gordon, 77–8, 117, 121, 132
Kennedy, John F., 12
Kieffer, Timothy, 118
King, Martin Luther, 14
Kleinsmith, Lewis, 43
Knowles, Lori P., 93–4
Kraft, Alison, 17–18, 32
Krushchev, Nikita, 12
Kubrick, Stanley, 13

Lavigne, Avril, 127
Leblond, Charles Philippe, 132
Lee, Harper, 14
Lemmon, Jack, 13
Lesage, Jean, 12
Ling, Victor, 21, 60
Loren, Sophia, 13
Lorenz, Egon, 17–18, 32
Loutit, John Freeman, 40

MacLaine, Shirley, 13
Macleod, J.J.R., 126–7
MacMurray, Fred, 13
Main, Joan M., 40
Mak, Tak Wah, 4, 53–6, 136
Mansbridge, Peter, 4
Marmont, Alberto, 107
Martin, Gail, 43–4
Mayer, Musa, 64
McBurney, Mike, 30, 49, 79
McCarthy, Jenny, 90
McCulloch, Jim, 27
McCulloch, Ona, 9, 27, 56
McEwan, Ian, 133
McEwen, Cheryl, 78, 121–2
McEwen, Rob, 78, 121
McEwen Centre for Regenerative Medicine, 78, 117, 120–2, 132
McQueen, Steve, 13
Medical Research Council, 29
Messner, Hans, 4, 42, 56–8, 107, 114
Metcalf, Donald, 40
Miller, Freda, 78–9, 92, 123
Miller, Rick, 57
Miller, Walter M., 14
Molson, Aaron, 105–7, 110–12
Molson, Jennifer, 105–14
Monroe, Marilyn, 13
Montand, Yves, 13
Morrison, Sean, 102–3
Mowat, Farley, 14
MS Society of Canada, 106

Nagy, Andras, 75–7
National Cancer Institute of Canada, 24, 29, 54, 61
National Institutes of Health, 29, 98
Naylor, David, 127–8, 132
Networks of Centres of Excellence, 65, 119
Nobel, Alfred, 129

Oak Ridge National Laboratory, 37
Obama, Barak, 76, 90, 115, 117, 124
Ontario Cancer Institute (OCI), 4, 9–10, 14, 16–18, 19–21, 23–30, 34–5, 37, 41–2, 44, 49–55, 58–61, 63–5, 66, 71–2, 74–7, 79, 107, 134, 136, 138
Ontario Cancer Treatment and Research Foundation, 29

Pablum, 132
Pasteur, Louis, 10, 125
Pasteur Institute, 25, 35
Penfield, Wilder, 126–7, 131
Peters, Vera, 35
Phillips, Bob, 29, 57, 60–1, 71, 77, 100, 136
Phillips, Gordon L., 59
Pierce, Barry, 43
Prehn, Richard T., 40
Prentice, Jim, 91
Presley, Elvis, 13
Princess Margaret Hospital, 3, 9, 42, 55, 57–8, 61, 70

radiation sickness, 15, 18, 116
Ragab, Abdul, 57
Ramalho-Santos, Miguel, 31–2
Richard, Maurice 'The Rocket,' 13
Richler, Mordecai, 23
Rider, Bill, 57
Rolling Stones, 14
Rossant, Janet, 74–6, 93
Rudnicki, Michael, 79–80, 132

Sabin, Albert, 16
Salk, Jonas, 15–16
Sauvageau, Guy, 66–7, 131
Scadden, David, 80–1, 128

Senn, John, 57
Sheinin, Rose, 28, 53
Shoichet, Molly, 70
Shumak, Ken, 58
Siminovitch, Lou, 21, 24–6, 28–9, 35–6, 50–1, 137
Singh, Sheila, 100, 119
Sipp, Douglas, 96–8
Smithies, Oliver, 44, 126
Spurgeon, David, 14
Stem Cell Network, 3, 65, 79–80, 116, 119, 132
Steptoe, Patrick, 128
Stevens, Leroy, 43
Stewart, Duncan, 117
Storb, Rainer, 40–2
Strauss, Evelyn, 37
Sutcliffe, Simon, 61–4

Temin, Howard, 53
Terry Fox Laboratory, 59, 72, 119
Terry Fox Research Institute, 60
Tetzlaff, Wolfram, 79
Thomas, E. Donnall, 18, 40–2, 95, 138
Till, Joyce, 20
Tisdall, Frederick, 132
Tremblay, Jacques, 118–19
Trentin, John J., 36
Tyrrell, Lorne, 131

van Bekkum, Dirk, 40
van der Kooy, Derek, 69–70

Wakefield, Andrew, 90
Watson, James, 16
Watson, Thomas, 14
Weiss, Samuel, 44, 68–70, 123
Weissman, Irving, 38–9, 128, 137
Whitmore, Gordon, 24, 28, 79
Wiesel, Torsten, 126
Wilkins, Maurice, 16
Willenbring, Holger, 31–2
Wilson, Edmund B., 31
Worton, Ron, 35, 65, 79–80, 116
Wright, Jim, 71

Yamanaka, Shinya, 75–7, 92, 131

Zandstra, Peter, 73–4, 120–1, 134
zur Hausen, Harald, 95